Medical Terminology

SHORT COURSE

Davi-Ellen Chabner, B.A., M.A.T.

Medical Terminology

A SHORT COURSE

THIRD EDITION

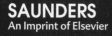

SAUNDERS
An Imprint of Elsevier

SAUNDERS
An Imprint of Elsevier

11830 Westline Industrial Drive
St. Louis, Missouri 63146

MEDICAL TERMINOLOGY: A SHORT COURSE   0-7216-9553-1

Previous editions copyrighted 1999, 1991

Library of Congress Cataloging-in-Publication Data

Chabner, Davi-Ellen.
    Medical terminology : a short course / Davi-Ellen Chabner.—3rd ed.
        p. ; cm.
    Includes index.
    ISBN 0-7216-9553-1
        1. Medicine—Terminology.   I. Title.
    [DNLM: 1. Terminology—Problems and Exercises.   W 15 C427m 2003]
    R123.C434 2003
    616'.0014—dc21

                                                2002075391

Publishing Director: Andrew Allen
Acquisitions Editor: Jeanne Wilke
Developmental Editor: Becky Swisher
Publishing Services Manager: Pat Joiner
Senior Designer: Mark A. Oberkrom
Designer: Judith A. Schmitt

TG/CTP

Printed in China

Last digit is the print number: 9   8   7   6   5   4   3

For
BENJAMIN OLIVER CHABNER
"Ben"
May 22, 2001

and

SAMUEL AUGUST THOMPSON
"Gust"
August 13, 2001

Both grandsons arrived during the writing of this book, and with Bebe and Solomon,
bring joy beyond compare to their "Mimi"!

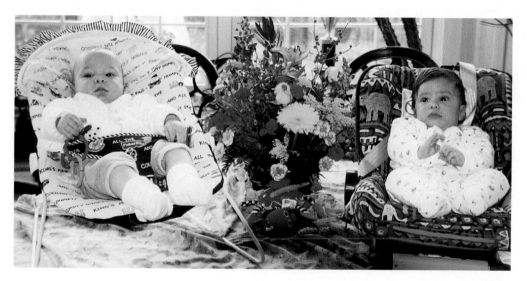

Thanksgiving 2001. Ben and Gust are well after precarious early days. See p. 121.

You will notice a striking change in the look of this new edition. I have revised all the figures in the text to bring you full-color images designed to enhance your ability to "see" medical terminology in action! This reflects my continuing belief that the best way to study and learn the medical language is to visualize it. New images of body parts (anatomy), disease conditions (pathology), and medical procedures will help you learn terminology by viewing it in its proper context.

The new images work together with a method that is fundamentally unaltered. I have preserved the simplicity, clarity, and practicality that characterized the two preceding editions. Thus the intent of *Medical Terminology: A Short Course,* third edition, is an introduction and overview of the medical language with emphasis on basic, essential information. Here are its important features:

- It is a self-teaching book with a workbook-text format that echoes the teaching method originally introduced in my more extensive text, *The Language of Medicine,* sixth edition. You learn by interaction and writing terms—answering questions, labeling diagrams, testing yourself with review sheets, and practicing pronunciation following guides in each chapter.

- It is easy to read and to understand. I have not assumed any background knowledge of biology or science. Explanations of terms are worded simply and clearly, and repetition reinforces learning throughout the text. Answers to exercise questions appear directly after the questions so that you may conveniently check your responses and learn from the printed answers.

- It is a valuable and comprehensive hospital and medical office reference guide. This feature of the book will be useful during your study and after completion of your course. Included are four appendixes. Appendix I, Body Systems, contains full-color images of each body system, labeled for easy reference to body parts. After each image are combining forms, terminology, pathology, and laboratory, diagnostic, and treatment procedures related to that system. Appendix II, Major Classes of Drugs, new to this edition, lists major classes of drugs and commonly prescribed examples in each class. Appendix III, Diagnostic Tests and Procedures, contains easy-to-understand explanations of radiological and nuclear medicine tests, as well as clinical procedures and laboratory tests in common use. Appendix IV, Abbreviations and Symbols, will help you reference practical and useful abbreviations you encounter on the job. The Glossaries of Medical Terms (a handy mini-dictionary of basic medical terms), Word Parts, and English → Spanish Terms should serve you well as you study and work in the medical field.

Throughout the text, you will find practical applications and medical vignettes illustrating terminology in the context of stories about patients. The *Instructor's Manual* contains classroom activities, quizzes, crossword puzzles, and more practical examples of case studies and medical reports. New to this edition is the inclusion of a CD-ROM, which contains pronunciation of all terms included on the pronunciation of terms lists in each chapter and additional practice in learning terminology.

Medical Terminology: A Short Course is exactly what you need to begin your medical career—in an office, hospital, or another medical-related setting. You can work at your own pace or use this book in a classroom setting with an instructor. The combination of visually reinforced learning *plus* easily accessible reference material will mean success for you in your allied health career!

Most of all, I hope this book excites your interest and enthusiasm for the medical language. I still have a strong passion for this subject, even after teaching and writing about it for over 25 years! Please communicate your comments and suggestions to me at MedDavi@aol.com.

Work hard, and have fun learning medical terminology!

Davi-Ellen Chabner

ACKNOWLEDGMENTS

Creating a medical terminology text is certainly not a solitary effort. It takes a crew! I am extremely fortunate to have a superb Acquisitions Editor, Maureen Pfeifer. Her intelligence, creativity, insight, and sound judgment are always on target and available to me. Thank you, Maureen, for your hard work and help!

I'm grateful for the staff at Elsevier Sciences for supporting and effectively marshaling the edition through its various stages. A special thank you to Becky Swisher, Associate Developmental Editor; Pat Joiner, Publishing Services Manager; Mark Oberkrom, Senior Designer; and Andrew Allen, Publishing Director. Jim Perkins skillfully created full-color images for this new edition, as he did for the sixth edition of *The Language of Medicine.* Esperanza Villanueva Joyce, EdD, CNS, RN, reviewed the Glossary of English → Spanish Terms, and I appreciated her suggestions. My friend, Luis Perelman, gave valuable advice as well.

The following teachers and students e-mailed comments and questions and provided invaluable advice for the current edition. They are Barbara Collignon, Cindy Correa, Geraud Dubois, Geraldine Giesker, William J. Martin, Heather Prutzman, Tom Owen, Mary Peterson, Gerald Selous, Eileen Steight, David Threefoot, Susan Webb, and Brandy Ziesemer. I appreciated every suggestion and look forward to hearing from all veteran and new users of this text.

As ever, I am grateful to my immediate family and especially to my husband, Bruce. His patient acceptance of my lifelong competing passion for the medical language makes everything possible.

Davi-Ellen Chabner

CONTENTS

Medical Terminology

A SHORT COURSE

BASIC WORD STRUCTURE

CHAPTER SECTIONS

CHAPTER OBJECTIVES

- To divide medical terms into component parts
- To analyze, pronounce, and spell medical terms using common combining forms, suffixes, and prefixes

I. WORD ANALYSIS

If you work in a medical setting, you use medical words every day. As a consumer and citizen, you hear medical terms in your doctor's office, read about health issues in the newspaper, and make daily decisions about your own health care and the health care of your family. Terms such as arthritis, electrocardiogram, hepatitis, and anemia describe conditions and tests that are familiar. Other medical words are more complicated, but as you work in this book, you will begin to understand them even if you have never studied biology or science.

Medical words are like individual jigsaw puzzles. Once you divide the terms into their component parts and learn the meaning of the individual parts, you can use that knowledge to understand many other new terms.

For example, the term HEMATOLOGY is divided into three parts:

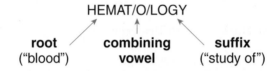

When you analyze a medical term, begin at the end of the word. The ending is called a **suffix.** All medical terms contain suffixes. The suffix in HEMATOLOGY is -LOGY, which means "study of." Now look at the beginning of the term. HEMAT- is the word **root.** The root gives the essential meaning of the term. The root HEMAT- means "blood."

The third part of this term, which is the letter O, has no meaning of its own but is an important connector between the root (HEMAT-) and the suffix (-LOGY). It is called a **combining vowel.** The letter O is the combining vowel usually found in medical terms.

Putting together the meaning of the suffix and the root, the term HEMATOLOGY means "the study of blood."

Here's another familiar medical term: ELECTROCARDIOGRAM. You probably know this term, often abbreviated as EKG or ECG. This is how you divide it into its parts:

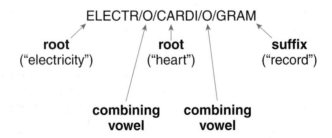

Start with the **suffix** at the end of the term. The suffix -GRAM means "a record."

Now look at the beginning of the term. ELECTR- is a word **root,** and it means "electricity."

This medical term has two roots. The second root is CARDI-, meaning "heart." Whenever you see CARDI- in other medical terms, you will know that it means "heart."

Read the meaning of medical terms from the suffix, back to the beginning of the term, then across. Thus the entire term means "record of the electricity in the heart." It is the electricity flowing within the heart that causes the heart muscle to contract, pumping blood throughout your body. The contraction and relaxation of heart muscle are called the heartbeat.

Notice the two combining vowels in ELECTROCARDIOGRAM. Looking for the O in medical terms will help you divide the term into its parts. One combining vowel (O) lies between roots (ELECTR- and CARDI-) and another between the root (CARDI-) and suffix (-GRAM).

The combining vowel *plus* the root is called a **combining form.** For example, there are *two* combining forms in the word ELECTROCARDIOGRAM. These combining forms are ELECTR/O, meaning "electricity," and CARDI/O, meaning "heart."

Notice how the following medical term is analyzed. Can you locate the two combining forms in this term?

GASTR/O/ENTER/O/LOGY

root	root	suffix
("stomach")	("intestines")	("study of")

The two combining forms are GASTR/O and ENTER/O. The entire word (reading from the suffix, back to the beginning of the term, and across) means "study of the stomach and the intestines." Here are other words that are divided into component parts:

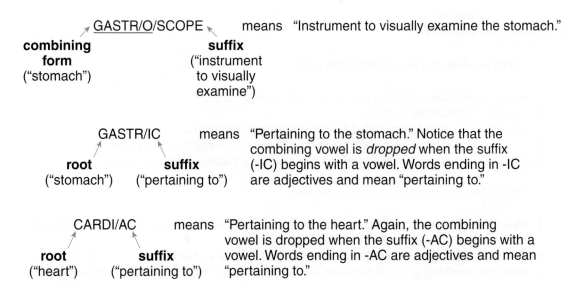

GASTR/O/SCOPE   means   "Instrument to visually examine the stomach."

combining form ("stomach")   **suffix** ("instrument to visually examine")

GASTR/IC   means   "Pertaining to the stomach." Notice that the combining vowel is *dropped* when the suffix (-IC) begins with a vowel. Words ending in -IC are adjectives and mean "pertaining to."

root ("stomach")   **suffix** ("pertaining to")

CARDI/AC   means   "Pertaining to the heart." Again, the combining vowel is dropped when the suffix (-AC) begins with a vowel. Words ending in -AC are adjectives and mean "pertaining to."

root ("heart")   **suffix** ("pertaining to")

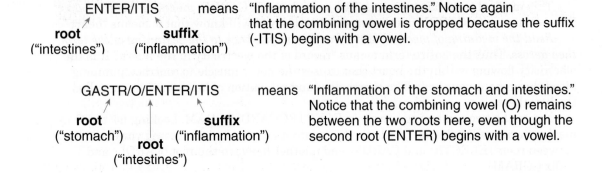

ENTER/ITIS   means   "Inflammation of the intestines." Notice again
that the combining vowel is dropped because the suffix
(-ITIS) begins with a vowel.

root   suffix
("intestines")   ("inflammation")

GASTR/O/ENTER/ITIS   means   "Inflammation of the stomach and intestines."
Notice that the combining vowel (O) remains
between the two roots here, even though the
second root (ENTER) begins with a vowel.

root   suffix
("stomach")   ("inflammation")
root
("intestines")

In addition to roots, suffixes, combining forms, and combining vowels, many medical terms have a word part attached to the *beginning* of the term. This is called a **prefix,** and it can change the meaning of a term in important ways. For example, watch what happens to the meaning of the following medical terms when the prefix changes:

SUB/gastr/ic   means   "Pertaining to *below* the stomach."

prefix
("below")

TRANS/gastr/ic   means   "Pertaining to *across* the stomach."

prefix
("across")

RETRO/gastr/ic   means   "Pertaining to *behind* the stomach."

prefix
("behind")

Let's **review** the important word parts:

1. **Root**—gives the essential *meaning* of the term.
2. **Suffix**—is the word *ending*.
3. **Prefix**—is a small part added to the *beginning* of a term.
4. **Combining vowel**—*connects* roots to suffixes and roots to other roots.
5. **Combining form**—is the combination of the *root* and *combining vowel*.

Some important rules to *remember* are:

1. *Read* the meaning of medical words from the suffix to the beginning of the word and then across.
2. *Drop* the combining vowel before a suffix that starts with a vowel.
3. *Keep* the combining vowel between word roots, even if the root begins with a vowel.

II. COMBINING FORMS, SUFFIXES, AND PREFIXES

Here is a list of combining forms, suffixes, and prefixes that are commonly found in medical terms. Write the meaning of the medical term on the line that is provided. There will be terms that are more difficult to understand even after you write the meanings of individual word parts. For these, more extensive explanations are given. To check your work, see the Glossary of Medical Terms, which contains meanings of all terms and can be found on p. 265.

In your study of medical terminology, you will find it helpful to practice writing terms and their meanings many times. Complete the Exercises in Section III, the Review in Section IV, and the Pronunciation of Terms list in Section V, as you begin your study of the medical language.

COMBINING FORMS

COMBINING FORM	MEANING	MEDICAL TERM	MEANING
aden/o	gland	adenoma _____ -OMA means "tumor" or "mass."	
		adenitis _____ -ITIS means "inflammation."	
arthr/o	joint	arthritis _____	
bi/o	life	biology _____ -LOGY means "study of."	
		biopsy _____ -OPSY means "to view." Living tissue is removed and viewed under a microscope.	
carcin/o	cancer, cancerous	carcinoma _____	
cardi/o	heart	cardiology_____	
cephal/o	head	cephalic _____ -IC means "pertaining to."	

cerebr/o   cerebrum, largest part of the brain

cerebral _____
-AL means "pertaining to." Figure 1-1 shows the cerebrum and some of its functions.

cerebrovascular accident (CVA) _____
-VASCULAR means "pertaining to blood vessels"; a CVA is commonly known as a stroke.

cyst/o   urinary bladder

cystoscope _____
-SCOPE means "instrument to visually examine." Figure 1-2 shows the urinary bladder and urinary tract. A cystoscope is placed through the urethra into the urinary bladder. See Figure 1-3.

FIGURE 1-1

The cerebrum and its functions.

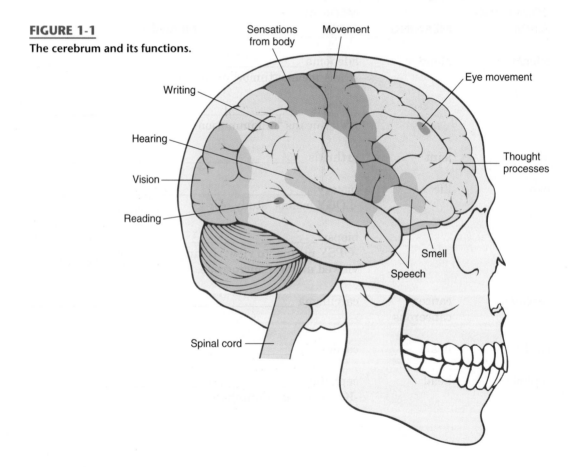

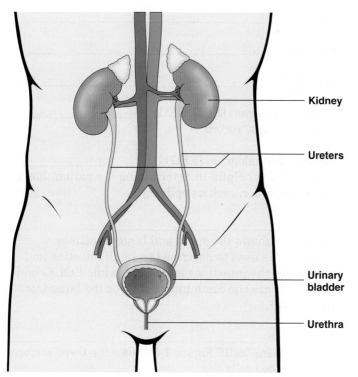

FIGURE 1-2
The urinary tract. (Modified from Chabner D-E: *The Language of Medicine,* ed 6, Philadelphia, 2001, WB Saunders.)

Kidney

Ureters

Urinary bladder

Urethra

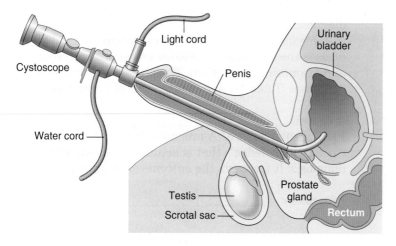

Light cord

Urinary bladder

Cystoscope

Penis

Water cord

Testis

Prostate gland

Scrotal sac

Rectum

FIGURE 1-3
Cystoscopy through the male urethra within the penis. (Modified from Chabner D-E: *The Language of Medicine,* ed 6, Philadelphia, 2001, WB Saunders.)

cyt/o	cell	cytology _____

dermat/o, derm/o	skin	dermatitis _____
		dermal _____

electr/o	electricity	electrocardiogram (ECG, EKG) _____

-GRAM means "record."

encephal/o	brain	electroencephalogram (EEG) _____

This record is helpful in determining if a patient has a seizure disorder, such as epilepsy.

enter/o	intestine (often the small intestine)	enteritis _____

Figure 1-4 shows the small and large intestines. ENTER/O is used to describe the small intestine and sometimes the intestines in general, while COL/O and COLON/O are the combining forms for the large intestine (colon).

erythr/o	red	erythrocyte _____

-CYTE means "cell." Figure 1-5 shows the three major types of blood cells.

gastr/o	stomach	gastroscopy _____

-SCOPY means "process of viewing."

gnos/o	knowledge	diagnosis _____

-SIS means "state of"; DIA- means "complete." A diagnosis is the complete knowledge gained after testing and examining the patient. The plural of diagnosis is diagnoses. Table 1-1 shows other plural formations.

prognosis _____

PRO- means "before." A prognosis is a prediction ("before knowledge") that is actually made after the diagnosis. It forecasts the outcome of treatment.

gynec/o	woman	gynecology _____

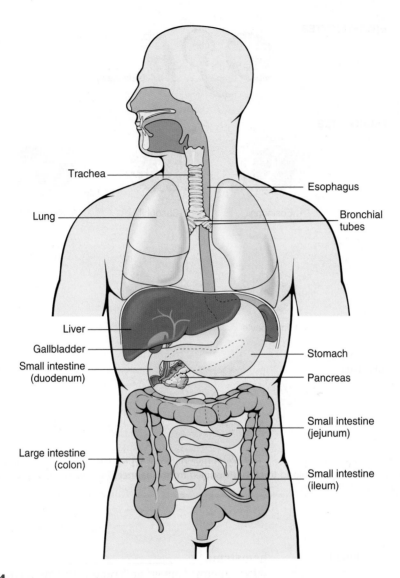

FIGURE 1-4

Location of the small and large intestines in the abdominal cavity. Note that the lungs, bronchial tubes, trachea, and esophagus are in the chest cavity. (Modified from Chabner D-E: *The Language of Medicine,* ed 6, Philadelphia, 2001, WB Saunders.)

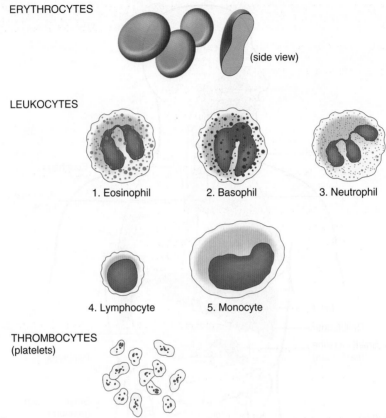

ERYTHROCYTES

(side view)

LEUKOCYTES

1. Eosinophil   2. Basophil   3. Neutrophil

4. Lymphocyte   5. Monocyte

THROMBOCYTES
(platelets)

FIGURE 1-5

Blood cells: *erythrocytes* (carry oxygen), *leukocytes* (five different types help fight disease), and *thrombocytes* or platelets (help blood to clot). (Modified from Chabner D-E: *The Language of Medicine,* ed 6, Philadelphia, 2001, WB Saunders.)

hemat/o, hem/o	blood	hematoma _____ -OMA means "mass" or "tumor." In this term, -oma indicates a mass or swelling containing blood. A hematoma is a bruise or black-and-blue mark.
		hemoglobin _____ -GLOBIN means "protein." Hemoglobin is the protein in red blood cells (erythrocytes) that helps carry oxygen in the blood.
hepat/o	liver	hepatitis _____

TABLE 1-1 ◆ Formation of Plurals

Consult the Glossary of Medical Terms for pronunciations of all terms.

1. Words ending in **a**, retain the **a** and add **e**:

SINGULAR	PLURAL	MEANING
verte**bra**	verte**brae**	Backbones
bur**sa**	bur**sae**	Sacs of fluid near a joint

2. Words ending in **is**, drop the **is** and add **es**:

SINGULAR	PLURAL	MEANING
diagno**sis**	diagno**ses**	Determinations of the nature and cause of diseases
psycho**sis**	psycho**ses**	Abnormal conditions of the mind

3. Words ending in **ex** or **ix**, drop the **ex** or **ix**, and add **ices**:

SINGULAR	PLURAL	MEANING
ap**ex**	ap**ices**	Pointed ends of organs
cort**ex**	cort**ices**	Outer parts of organs
var**ix**	var**ices**	Enlarged, swollen veins

4. Words ending in **on**, drop the **on** and add **a**:

SINGULAR	PLURAL	MEANING
gangli**on**	gangli**a**	Groups of nerve cells; benign cysts near a joint (such as the wrist)

5. Words ending in **um**, drop the **um** and add **a**:

SINGULAR	PLURAL	MEANING
bacteri**um**	bacteri**a**	Types of one-celled organisms
ov**um**	ov**a**	Egg cells

6. Words ending in **us**, drop the **us** and add **i***:

SINGULAR	PLURAL	MEANING
bronch**us**	bronch**i**	Tubes leading from the windpipe to the lungs
calcul**us**	calcul**i**	Stones

*Exceptions to this rule are viruses and sinuses.

lapar/o	abdomen (area between the chest and hip)	laparotomy _____ -TOMY means "incision" (to cut into). An exploratory laparotomy is a large incision of the abdominal wall made to inspect abdominal organs for evidence of disease. Another combining form for abdomen is ABDOMIN/O as in abdominal.
leuk/o	white	leukocyte _____ Figure 1-5 shows five different types of leukocytes.

nephr/o	kidney	nephrectomy _____ -ECTOMY means "to cut out," an excision or resection of an organ or part of the body.
neur/o	nerve	neurology _____
onc/o	tumor	oncologist _____ -IST means "a specialist."
ophthalm/o	eye	ophthalmoscope _____ Figure 1-6 shows an ophthalmologist examining a patient with an ophthalmoscope.
oste/o	bone	osteoarthritis _____ Figure 1-7 shows a normal knee joint and a knee joint with osteoarthritis. Degenerative changes and loss of cartilage occur. Inflammation of the joint membrane occurs late in the disease.
path/o	disease	pathologist _____ A pathologist is a medical doctor who views biopsy samples to make a diagnosis and examines a dead body (in an autopsy) to determine the cause of death. AUT- means "self," and -OPSY means "to view." Thus, an autopsy is an opportunity to see for oneself what has happened to the patient to cause his or her death.
psych/o	mind	psychosis _____ -OSIS means "abnormal condition." This is a serious mental condition in which the patient loses touch with reality.
ren/o	kidney	renal _____ Sometimes there are *two* combining forms for the same part of the body. One comes from Latin, and the other from Greek (REN- is the Latin root meaning "kidney," and NEPHR- is the Greek root). The Greek root is used to describe abnormal conditions and procedures, whereas the Latin root is used with -AL, meaning "pertaining to."
rhin/o	nose	rhinitis _____

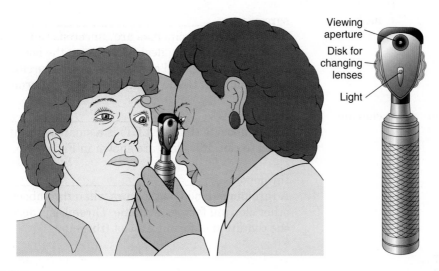

Viewing aperture
Disk for changing lenses
Light

FIGURE 1-6

The ophthalmoscope. It allows the *ophthalmologist* to view the outer and inner areas of the eye. (Modified from Chabner D-E: *The Language of Medicine,* ed 6, Philadelphia, 2001, WB Saunders.)

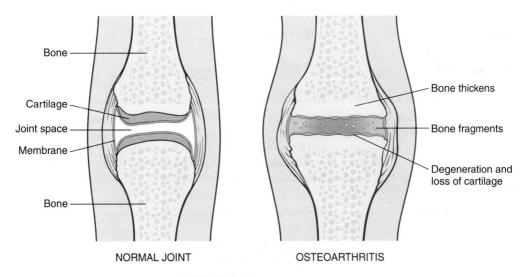

Bone
Cartilage
Joint space
Membrane
Bone

Bone thickens
Bone fragments
Degeneration and loss of cartilage

NORMAL JOINT   OSTEOARTHRITIS

FIGURE 1-7

Normal joint with osteoarthritis.

| sarc/o | flesh | sarcoma _____ |

Sarcomas and carcinomas are cancerous tumors. Sarcomas grow from the "fleshy" tissues of the body, such as muscle, fat, bone, and cartilage, whereas carcinomas arise from skin tissue and the linings of internal organs.

| thromb/o | clotting | thrombocyte _____ |

A thrombocyte (PLATELET) is a small cell that helps blood to clot. Platelets are shown in Figure 1-5.

thrombosis_____

A thrombus (blood clot) occurs when thrombocytes and other clotting factors combine. Thrombosis describes the condition of forming a clot (thrombus).

SUFFIXES

SUFFIX	MEANING	MEDICAL TERM	MEANING
-al	pertaining to	neural _____	
-algia	pain	arthralgia _____	
-cyte	cell	leukocyte _____	
-ectomy	removal, excision	gastrectomy _____	
-emia	blood condition	leukemia _____	

Large numbers of immature, cancerous cells are found in the bloodstream and bone marrow (inner part of bone that makes blood cells).

| -globin | protein | hemoglobin _____ | |
| -gram | record | arthrogram _____ | |

This is an x-ray record of a joint.

| -ic | pertaining to | gastric _____ | |
| -ism | condition, process | hyperthyroidism _____ | |

HYPER- means "excessive." The thyroid gland is in the neck. It secretes (makes) a hormone called thyroxine, which helps cells burn food to release energy. See Figure 1-8.

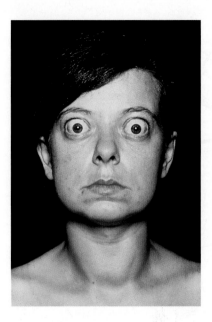

FIGURE 1-8

Hyperthyroidism. The thyroid gland produces too much hormone and causes symptoms such as rapid pulse, nervousness, excessive sweating, and swelling of tissue behind the eyeball. (Modified from Seidel H et al: *Mosby's Guide to Physical Examination,* ed 4, St. Louis, 1998, Mosby.)

TABLE 1-2 ▸ Terms Using -LOGY (Study Of)	
cardiology	Study of the heart
dermatology	Study of the skin
endocrinology	Study of the endocrine glands
gastroenterology	Study of the stomach and intestines
gynecology	Study of women and women's disease
hematology	Study of the blood
neurology	Study of the nerves and the brain and spinal cord
oncology	Study of tumors (cancerous or malignant diseases)
ophthalmology	Study of the eye
pathology	Study of disease
psychology	Study of the mind and mental disorders
rheumatology	Study of joint diseases (RHEUMAT/O means "flow or watery discharge," which was once thought to cause aches and pains, especially in joints.)

-itis	inflammation	gastroenteritis _____
-logist	specialist in the study of	neurologist _____
-logy	study of	nephrology _____

See Table 1-2 for a list of other terms using -LOGY.

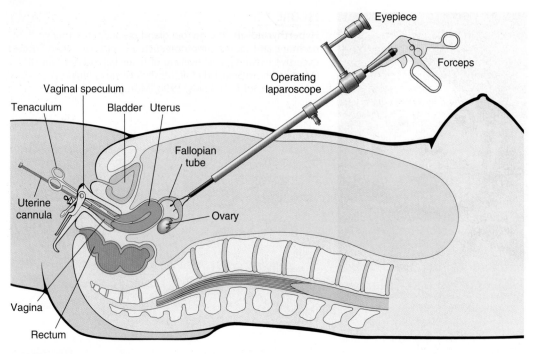

FIGURE 1-9

Laparoscopy for tubal ligation (interruption of the continuity of the fallopian tubes) as a means of preventing future pregnancy. The *tenaculum* keeps the vaginal cavity open. The *uterine cannula* is a tube placed into the uterus to move the uterus during the procedure. *Forceps,* placed through the laparoscope, are used for grasping or manipulating tissue. (Modified from Chabner D-E: *The Language of Medicine,* ed 6, Philadelphia, 2001, WB Saunders.)

-oma	tumor, mass	hepatoma _____
-opsy	to view	biopsy _____
-osis	abnormal condition	nephrosis _____
-scope	instrument to visually examine	gastroscope _____
-scopy	process of visual examination	laparoscopy _____ Small incisions are made near the navel, and tubes are inserted into the abdomen for viewing organs and doing procedures such as tying off the fallopian tubes. See Figure 1-9.

FIGURE 1-10

Arthroscopy of the knee. An arthroscope is used in the diagnosis of pathological changes. (Modified from Lewis SM, Collier IC, Heitkemper MM: *Medical-Surgical Nursing: Assessment and Management of Clinical Problems,* ed 4, St. Louis, 1996, Mosby.)

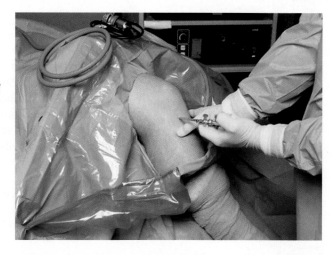

arthroscopy _____
See Figure 1-10.

-sis   state of   prognosis _____

-tomy   process of cutting, incision   neurotomy _____

PREFIXES

PREFIXES	MEANING	MEDICAL TERM	MEANING
a-, an-	no, not	anemia _____ Literally, *anemia* means a condition of "no blood." Actually, it is a decrease in the number of red blood cells or a decrease in their ability to carry oxygen because of less hemoglobin, a protein that helps carry oxygen in red blood cells.	
aut-	self	autopsy _____ Viewing and examining a dead body with one's own (self) eyes.	
dia-	complete, through	diagnosis _____	

dys-	bad, painful, difficult, abnormal	dysentery _____ The suffix -Y means condition or process.
endo-	within	endocrine glands _____ -CRIN/O means "to secrete" (to form and give off). Examples of endocrine glands are the thyroid gland, pituitary gland, adrenal glands, ovaries, and testes. All these glands secrete hormones within the body and *into* the bloodstream.
exo-	outside	exocrine glands_____ Examples of exocrine glands are sweat, tear, and mammary (breast) glands that secrete substances to the *outside* of the body.
hyper-	excessive, more than normal	hyperglycemia _____ GLYC/O- means "sugar." Hyperglycemia is also known as diabetes mellitus. *Mellitus* means "sweet."
hypo-	below, less than normal	hypodermic _____ A hypodermic syringe (an instrument for injecting or withdrawing fluid) is placed under the skin. See Figure 1-11. hypoglycemia _____

FIGURE 1-11

A hypodermic syringe inserted under the skin.

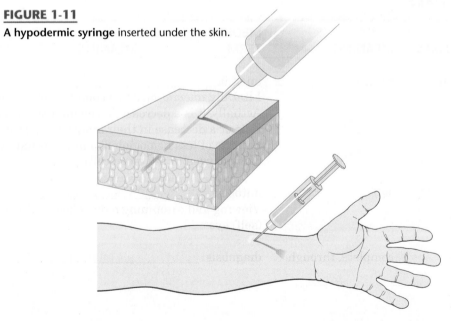

pro-	before	prognosis _____
re-	back	resection _____
		-SECTION means "to cut into an organ," but resection means "to cut an organ out in the sense of cutting back or away." The Latin *resectio* means "a trimming or pruning."
retro-	behind	retrogastric _____
sub-	under, below	subhepatic _____
trans-	across, through	transurethral _____
		The urethra is the tube that leads from the urinary bladder to the outside of the body. See Figure 1-2.

III. EXERCISES

These exercises give you practice writing and understanding the terms presented in Section II. An important part of your work is to *check your answers* with the answer key given directly after the exercises on p. 20. If you can't answer a question, then *please* look at the answer key and *copy* the correct answer. You may want to photocopy some of the exercises before you complete them so that you can practice doing them many times.

A. **Using slashes, divide the following terms into their component parts and give the meaning for the whole term:**

1. adenoma _____

2. arthritis _____

3. enteric _____

4. encephalitis _____

5. dermatosis _____

6. oncologist _____

7. arthroscope _____

8. cerebral _____

9. cardiology _____

10. transhepatic _____

11. cephalic _____

◆ **ANSWER KEY**
1. aden/oma—tumor of a gland
2. arthr/itis—inflammation of a joint
3. enter/ic—pertaining to the intestines
4. encephal/itis—inflammation of the brain
5. dermat/osis—abnormal condition of the skin
6. onc/o/logist—specialist in the study of tumors
7. arthr/o/scope—instrument to visually examine a joint
8. cerebr/al—pertaining to the brain or cerebrum, its largest part
9. cardi/o/logy—study of the heart
10. trans/hepat/ic—pertaining to across or through the liver
11. cephal/ic—pertaining to the head

B. **Complete the following medical terms:**

1. _____ gastric   pertaining to under the stomach

2. gastr _____   pain in the stomach

3. gastr _____   inflammation of the stomach

4. _____ gastric   pertaining to across the stomach

5. gastr _____   process of visually examining the stomach

6. _____ gastric   pertaining to behind the stomach

7. gastr _____   instrument for visually examining the stomach

8. gastr _____   study of the stomach and intestines

9. gastr _____   excision (removal) of the stomach

10. gastr _____   incision (to cut into) of the stomach

◆ **ANSWER KEY**

1. subgastric	6. retrogastric
2. gastralgia	7. gastroscope
3. gastritis	8. gastroenterology
4. transgastric	9. gastrectomy
5. gastroscopy	10. gastrotomy

C. What part of the body do the following medical terms refer to? Give the meaning for each term.

1. adenoma _____

2. enteritis _____

3. arthrosis _____

4. cerebrovascular accident _____
   (VASCULAR means "pertaining to blood vessels"; a cerebrovascular accident is also known as a *stroke,* or *CVA*)

5. dermatitis _____

6. encephalitis _____

7. renal _____

8. osteitis _____

9. nephritis _____

10. electroencephalogram _____

11. rhinitis _____

12. laparotomy _____

13. ophthalmology _____

14. hepatoma _____

◆ **ANSWER KEY**
1. gland—tumor of a gland
2. intestine (usually the small intestine)—inflammation of the intestine
3. joint—abnormal condition of a joint
4. brain (cerebrum)—accident pertaining to the blood vessels of the brain
5. skin—inflammation of the skin
6. brain—inflammation of the brain
7. kidney—pertaining to a kidney
8. bone—inflammation of bone
9. kidney—inflammation of a kidney
10. brain—record of electricity in the brain
11. nose—inflammation of the nose
12. abdomen—incision of the abdomen
13. eye—study of the eye
14. liver—tumor of the liver

D. Using slashes, divide each of the following terms into its component parts and give the meaning of the whole term:

1. nephrectomy _____

2. neuritis _____

3. oncology _____

4. gastralgia _____

5. hepatitis _____

6. endocrinology _____
Endocrine glands produce hormones; examples are the thyroid gland in the neck, the pituitary gland at the base of the brain, the ovaries in the female, and the testes in the male.

7. osteoarthritis _____

8. psychology _____

9. dermatosis _____

10. gynecology _____

11. sarcoma _____

12. carcinoma _____

13. transurethral _____

14. ophthalmoscope _____

15. dermal _____

16. hemoglobin _____

◆ **ANSWER KEY**

1. nephr/ectomy—removal or excision of a kidney
2. neur/itis—inflammation of a nerve
3. onc/o/logy—study of tumors
4. gastr/algia—pain in the stomach
5. hepat/itis—inflammation of the liver
6. endo/crin/o/logy—study of the endocrine glands (glands that secrete hormones into the bloodstream)
7. oste/o/arthr/itis—inflammation of bones and joints
8. psych/o/logy—study of the mind
9. dermat/osis—abnormal condition of the skin
10. gynec/o/logy—study of women (disorders of the female reproductive organs)
11. sarc/oma—tumor (cancerous) of flesh tissue
12. carcin/oma—cancerous tumor (of skin cells or cells that line the internal organs)
13. trans/urethr/al—pertaining to through the urethra (tube that leads from the bladder to the outside of the body)
14. ophthalm/o/scope—instrument to visually examine the eye
15. derm/al—pertaining to the skin
16. hem/o/globin—protein of the blood (carries oxygen and found in red blood cells)

E. Complete the following medical terms:

1. _____ cyte   A **red** blood cell; these cells carry oxygen to all parts of the body.

2. _____ cyte   A **white** blood cell; these cells help to fight disease.

3. _____ cyte   A **clotting** cell; these cells help your blood to clot and are also called *platelets*.

4. _____ gnosis   A state of **complete** knowledge; what your doctor tells you about your condition after testing and examination.

5. _____ thyroidism   A condition of **excessive** production of hormone from the thyroid gland.

6. _____ thyroidism   A condition of **decreased** production of hormone from the thyroid gland.

7. leuk _____   A **blood condition** of too many white blood cells; the cells are cancerous.

8. _____ logy   Study of **nerves** and nervous disorders.

9. _____ oma   Tumor of the **liver.**

10. _____ logy   Study of **disease.**

◆ **ANSWER KEY**
1. erythrocyte	6. hypothyroidism
2. leukocyte	7. leukemia
3. thrombocyte	8. neurology
4. diagnosis	9. hepatoma
5. hyperthyroidism	10. pathology

F. Use a slash to identify the suffix in each of the following, and give the meaning of the entire term:

1. osteotomy _____

2. rhinitis _____

3. neuralgia _____

4. nephrosis _____

5. adenectomy _____

6. cerebral _____

7. arthrogram _____

8. laparoscopy _____

9. laparotomy _____

10. hepatitis _____

11. cephalalgia _____

◆ **ANSWER KEY**
1. osteo/tomy (process of cutting bone)
2. rhin/itis (inflammation of the nose)
3. neur/algia (pain of a nerve)
4. nephr/osis (abnormal condition of the kidney)
5. aden/ectomy (removal of a gland)
6. cerebr/al (pertaining to the cerebrum, the largest part of the brain)
7. arthro/gram (record, x-ray, of a joint)
8. laparo/scopy (visual examination of the abdomen)
9. laparo/tomy (incision of the abdomen)
10. hepat/itis (inflammation of the liver)
11. cephal/algia or often shortened to ceph/algia (pain in the head)

G. **Give the meaning for the underlined term in each of the following sentences:**

1. An oncologist treats patients who have sarcomas and carcinomas. _____

_____

2. After explaining Mr. Green's diagnosis to him and outlining the plan of treatment, Dr. Jones assured him that the <u>prognosis</u> was hopeful. _____

_____

3. Seventy-five-year-old Ms. Stein has constant pain in her knees and hips. Her doctor tells her that she has degeneration of her joints and recommends that she take aspirin and other drugs to reduce the discomfort caused by her <u>osteoarthritis</u>.

_____

4. <u>Thrombosis</u> is a serious condition that can lead to blockage of blood vessels. If the blockage stops blood from reaching body cells, those cells die because they are deprived of the food and oxygen that are carried by the blood._____

_____

5. A <u>pathologist</u> is the medical doctor who specializes in examining biopsy samples and performing autopsies. _____

6. <u>Hyperglycemia</u> can result from a lack of insulin (hormone) secretion from the pancreas (an endocrine gland near the stomach). Without insulin, sugar remains in the blood and cannot enter body cells. _____

_____

7. A patient with a <u>psychosis</u> loses touch with the real world and displays abnormal behavior. _____

8. A doctor uses a cystoscope to perform a <u>cystoscopy</u>. _____

9. A <u>laparotomy</u> may be necessary to determine the spread of disease in the abdomen.

   _____

10. The doctor used a <u>laparoscope</u> to cut and tie off Ms. Smith's fallopian tubes so that

    she couldn't become pregnant. _____

    _____

11. Symptoms of <u>hyperthyroidism</u> may include an enlarged thyroid gland, speeding up

    of bodily processes, and protruding eyeballs (exophthalmos). _____

    _____

12. Mr. Paul had a partial <u>resection</u> of his stomach as treatment for his gastric

    adenocarcinoma. _____

13. <u>Leukemia</u> is diagnosed by looking at a blood sample or taking a bone marrow

    biopsy. _____

14. A <u>transurethral</u> resection of the prostate gland is a treatment for the overdevelop-

    ment of that gland, which is located below the bladder in males. _____

    _____

15. When Sally returned from her trip to Mexico, she experienced abdominal pain,

    fever, and severe diarrhea. Her doctor told her she was suffering from <u>dysentery</u>.

    _____

16. The cerebral blood clot discovered during Mr. Smith's <u>autopsy</u> confirmed his doctor's

    diagnosis of CVA. _____

    _____

◆ **ANSWER KEY**
1. specialist in the study of tumors
2. prediction about the outcome of treatment (literally, "before knowledge")
3. inflammation of bones and joints
4. abnormal condition of clotting or clot formation
5. specialist in the study of disease
6. blood condition of too much sugar
7. abnormal condition of the mind
8. process of visual examination of the urinary bladder
9. incision of the abdomen
10. instrument to visually examine the abdomen
11. condition of too much thyroid hormone
12. removal, excision
13. cancerous condition of white blood cells
14. across (through) the urethra
15. painful intestines
16. examination of a dead body

H. Refer to Table 1-1 to form the plurals of the following terms:

1. psychosis _____

2. ovum _____

3. vertebra _____

4. bronchus _____

5. spermatozoon _____

6. apex _____

◆ **ANSWER KEY**
1. psychoses (drop **-is** and add **-es**)
2. ova (drop **-um** and add **-a**)
3. vertebra (add **-e**)
4. bronchi (drop **-us** and add **-i**)
5. spermatozoa (drop **-on** and add **-a**)
6. apices (drop **-ex** and add **-ices**)

I. Circle the term that best completes the meaning of the sentences in the following medical vignettes:

1. Selma ate a spicy meal at an Indian restaurant. Later that night she experienced **(osteoarthritis, dermatitis, gastroenteritis).** Fortunately, the cramping and diarrhea subsided by morning.

2. Christina was feeling very sluggish, both physically and mentally. Her hair seemed coarse, she had noticed weight gain in the past weeks, and she had hot and cold intolerance, never really feeling comfortable. Her internist referred her to a specialist, a(an) **(gynecologist, endocrinologist, pathologist).** The physician did a blood test that revealed low levels of a hormone from a gland in her neck. The diagnosis of **(hypothyroidism, hyperthyroidism, psychosis)** was thus made and proper treatment prescribed.

3. Dr. Fischer examined the lump in Bruno's thigh. A special imaging technique using magnetic waves and radio signals (an MRI scan) revealed a suspicious mass in the soft connective tissue **(hematoma, carcinoma, sarcoma).** The doctor then suggested a(an) **(prognosis, biopsy, autopsy)** to determine if the mass was malignant.

4. On her seventh birthday, Susie fell down during her birthday party. Her mother noticed bruises on Susie's knees and elbows that seemed to come up "over night." Her pediatrician ordered a blood test that demonstrated lowered thrombocyte count and an elevated **(leukocyte, erythrocyte, platelet)** count at 30,000 cells. Susie was referred to a(an) **(dermatologist, nephrologist, oncologist),** who made a diagnosis of acute **(hepatitis, anemia, leukemia).**

5. When Mr. Saluto collapsed and died while eating dinner, the family requested a(an) **(laparotomy, gastroscopy, autopsy)** to determine the cause of death. The **(hematologist, pathologist, gastroenterologist)** discovered that Mr. Saluto had died of a **(cardiovascular accident, dysentery, cerebrovascular accident),** otherwise known as a stroke.

◆ **ANSWER KEY**
1. gastroenteritis
2. endocrinologist, hypothyroidism
3. sarcoma, biopsy
4. leukocyte, oncologist, leukemia
5. autopsy, pathologist, cerebrovascular accident

IV. REVIEW

Here's your chance to test your understanding of all the **combining forms, suffixes,** and **prefixes** that you have studied in this chapter. Write the meaning of each term in the space provided and *check* your answers with the answer key at the end of each list!

COMBINING FORMS

COMBINING FORM	MEANING	COMBINING FORM	MEANING
1. aden/o		17. gnos/o	
2. arthr/o		18. gynec/o	
3. bi/o		19. hemat/o, hem/o	
4. carcin/o		20. hepat/o	
5. cardi/o		21. lapar/o	
6. cephal/o		22. leuk/o	
7. cerebr/o		23. nephr/o	
8. cyst/o		24. neur/o	
9. cyt/o		25. onc/o	
10. dermat/o, derm/o		26. ophthalm/o	
11. electr/o		27. oste/o	
12. encephal/o		28. path/o	
13. enter/o		29. psych/o	
14. erythr/o		30. rhin/o	
15. gastr/o		31. sarc/o	
16. glyc/o		32. thromb/o	

SUFFIXES

SUFFIX	MEANING	SUFFIX	MEANING
1. -al	_____	10. -logist	_____
2. -algia	_____	11. -logy	_____
3. -cyte	_____	12. -oma	_____
4. -ectomy	_____	13. -opsy	_____
5. -emia	_____	14. -osis	_____
6. -globin	_____	15. -scope	_____
7. -ic	_____	16. -scopy	_____
8. -ism	_____	17. -sis	_____
9. -itis	_____	18. -tomy	_____

PREFIXES

PREFIX	MEANING	PREFIX	MEANING
1. a-, an-	_____	8. hypo-	_____
2. aut-	_____	9. pro-	_____
3. dia-	_____	10. re-	_____
4. dys-	_____	11. retro-	_____
5. endo-	_____	12. sub-	_____
6. exo-	_____	13. trans-	_____
7. hyper-	_____		

COMBINING FORMS

◆ **ANSWER KEY**

1. gland	17. knowledge
2. joint	18. woman, female
3. life	19. blood
4. cancerous	20. liver
5. heart	21. abdomen
6. head	22. white
7. cerebrum	23. kidney
8. urinary bladder	24. nerve
9. cell	25. tumor
10. skin	26. eye
11. electricity	27. bone
12. brain	28. disease
13. intestines	29. mind
14. red	30. nose
15. stomach	31. flesh
16. sugar	32. clot

SUFFIXES

◆ **ANSWER KEY**

1. pertaining to	11. study of
2. pain	12. tumor, mass
3. cell	13. to view
4. removal; excision	14. abnormal condition
5. blood condition	15. instrument to visually examine
6. protein	16. process of visual examination
7. pertaining to	17. state of
8. condition; process	18. process of cutting; incision
9. inflammation	
10. specialist in the study of	

PREFIXES

◆ **ANSWER KEY**

1. no, not	7. too much, above
2. self	8. below, too little, deficient
3. complete	9. before
4. bad, painful, difficult, abnormal	10. back
5. within	11. behind
6. out, outside	12. under, below
	13. across, through

V. PRONUNCIATION OF TERMS

The terms that you have learned in this chapter are presented here with their pronunciations. The capitalized letters in boldface are the accented syllable. Pronounce each word out loud, then write the meaning in the space provided.

TERM	PRONUNCIATION	MEANING
adenitis	ad-eh-**NI**-tis	
adenoma	ah-deh-**NO**-mah	
anemia	ah-**NE**-me-ah	
arthralgia	ar-**THRAL**-jah	
arthritis	ar-**THRI**-tis	
arthrogram	**AR**-thro-gram	
arthroscope	**AR**-thro-skop	
arthroscopy	ar-**THROS**-ko-pe	
autopsy	**AW**-top-se	
biology	bi-**OL**-o-je	
biopsy	**BI**-op-se	
carcinoma	kar-sih-**NO**-mah	
cardiac	**KAR**-de-ak	
cardiology	kar-de-**OL**-o-je	
cephalic	seh-**FAL**-ik	
cerebral	seh-**RE**-bral	
cerebrovascular accident	seh-re-bro-**VAS**-ku-lar **AK**-sih-dent	

cystoscope	**SIS**-to-skop
cystoscopy	sis-**TOS**-ko-pe
cytology	si-**TOL**-o-je
dermatitis	der-mah-**TI**-tis
dermal	**DER**-mal
dermatosis	der-mah-**TO**-sis
diagnosis	di-ag-**NO**-sis
dysentery	**DIS**-en-teh-re
electrocardiogram	e-lek-tro-**KAR**-de-o-gram
electroencephalogram	e-lek-tro-en-**SEF**-ah-lo-gram
endocrine glands	**EN**-do-krin glanz
endocrinology	en-do-krih-**NOL**-o-je
enteritis	en-teh-**RI**-tis
erythrocyte	eh-**RITH**-ro-site
exocrine glands	**EK**-so-krin glanz
gastrectomy	gas-**TREK**-to-me
gastric	**GAS**-trik
gastritis	gas-**TRI**-tis
gastroenteritis	gas-tro-en-teh-**RI**-tis
gastroenterology	gas-tro-en-ter-**OL**-o-je
gastroscope	**GAS**-tro-skop
gastroscopy	gas-**TROS**-ko-pe

gastrotomy	gas-**TROT**-o-me	
gynecologist	gi-neh-**KOL**-o-jist	
gynecology	gi-neh-**KOL**-o-je	
hematoma	**he**-mah-**TO**-mah	
hemoglobin	**HE**-mo-glo-bin	
hepatitis	hep-ah-**TI**-tis	
hepatoma	hep-ah-**TO**-mah	
hyperglycemia	hi-per-gli-**SE**-me-ah	
hyperthyroidism	hi-per-**THI**-royd-izm	
hypodermic	hi-po-**DER**-mik	
hypoglycemia	hi-po-gli-**SE**-me-ah	
hypothyroidism	hi-po-**THI**-royd-izm	
laparoscopy	lap-ah-**ROS**-ko-pe	
laparotomy	lap-ah-**ROT**-o-me	
leukemia	lu-**KE**-me-ah	
leukocyte	**LU**-ko-site	
nephrectomy	neh-**FREK**-to-me	
nephrology	neh-**FROL**-o-je	
nephrosis	neh-**FRO**-sis	
neural	**NU**-ral	
neuralgia	nu-**RAL**-jah	
neuritis	nu-**RI**-tis	

neurology	nur-**ROL**-o-je _____
neurotomy	nur-**ROT**-o-me _____
oncologist	ong-**KOL**-o-jist _____
ophthalmoscope	of-**THAL**-mo-skop _____
osteitis	os-te-**I**-tis _____
osteoarthritis	os-te-o-ar-**THRI**-tis _____
pathologist	pah-**THOL**-o-jist _____
platelet	**PLAT**-let _____
prognosis	prog-**NO**-sis _____
psychosis	si-**KO**-**sis** _____
renal	**RE**-nal _____
resection	re-**SEK**-shun _____
retrogastric	reh-tro-**GAS**-trik _____
rhinitis	ri-**NI**-tis _____
rhinotomy	ri-**NOT**-o-me _____
sarcoma	sar-**KO**-mah _____
subgastric	sub-**GAS**-trik _____
subhepatic	sub-heh-**PAT**-ik _____
thrombocyte	**THROM**-bo-site _____
thrombosis	throm-**BO**-sis _____
transgastric	trans-**GAS**-trik _____
transurethral	trans-u-**RE**-thral _____

VI. PRACTICAL APPLICATIONS

Match the **procedure** in Column I with the **diagnosis** that it treats (or helps to diagnose) in Column II. Can you also name the physician who would perform each procedure?

COLUMN I	COLUMN II
PROCEDURE	*DIAGNOSIS*

1. nephrectomy   _____   a. leukemia

2. thyroid gland resection   _____   b. urinary bladder carcinoma

3. electroencephalogram   _____   c. adenocarcinoma of an endocrine gland in the neck

4. below-knee amputation (resection)   _____   d. stomach ulcer

5. electrocardiogram   _____   e. seizure disorder (epilepsy)

6. gastroscopy   _____   f. osteogenic sarcoma (bone cancer)

7. bone marrow biopsy   _____   g. renal cell carcinoma

8. cystoscopy   _____   h. heart attack

◆ **ANSWER KEY**

1. g (urologist)
2. c (head and neck surgeon— an endocrinologist is an internist, not a surgeon)
3. e (neurologist)
4. f (orthopedist)
5. h (cardiologist)
6. d (gastroenterologist)
7. a (oncologist)
8. b (urologist)

ORGANIZATION OF THE BODY

CHAPTER SECTIONS

CHAPTER OBJECTIVES

- To name the body systems and their functions
- To identify body cavities and specific organs within them
- To list the divisions of the back
- To identify three planes of the body
- To analyze, pronounce, and spell new terms related to organs and tissues in the body

I. BODY SYSTEMS

All the parts of your body are composed of individual units called **cells.** Muscle, nerve, skin (epithelial), and bone cells are some examples.

Similar cells grouped together are **tissues.** Groups of muscle cells are muscle tissue, and groups of epithelial cells are epithelial tissue.

Collections of different tissues working together are called **organs.** An organ, such as the stomach, has different tissues, such as muscle, epithelial (lining of internal organs and outer layer of skin cells), and nerve, that help the organ function.

Groups of organs working together are the **systems** of the body. The digestive system, for example, includes organs such as the mouth, throat, esophagus, stomach, and intestines that bring food into the body and deliver it to the bloodstream.

There are eleven systems of the body, and each plays an important role in the way the body works.

The **circulatory system** (the heart, blood, and blood vessels such as arteries, veins, and capillaries) transports blood throughout the body. The **lymphatic system** includes lymph vessels and nodes that carry a clear fluid called lymph. Lymph contains white blood cells called lymphocytes that fight against disease and play an important role in immunity.

The **digestive system** brings food into the body and breaks it down so that it can enter the bloodstream. Food that cannot be broken down is then removed from the body at the end of the system.

The **endocrine system,** which is made up of glands, sends chemical messengers called *hormones* into the blood to act on other glands and organs.

The **female and male reproductive systems** produce the cells that join to form the embryo, fetus, and infant. Male (testis) and female (ovary) sex organs produce hormones as well.

The **musculoskeletal system,** including muscles, bones, joints, and connective tissues, supports the body and allows it to move.

The **nervous system** carries electrical messages to and from the brain and spinal cord.

The **respiratory system** controls breathing, a process in which air enters and leaves the body.

The **skin and sense organ system,** including the skin and eyes and ears, receives messages from the environment and sends them to the brain.

The **urinary system** produces urine and sends it out of the body through the kidneys, ureters, bladder, and urethra.

Appendix I, at the back of the book, contains diagrams of each body system along with combining forms for body parts, examples of terminology and pathology, and laboratory tests and diagnostic and treatment procedures. Appendix II is a reference for major classes of drugs and examples of common drugs in each class. Appendix III is a complete list of diagnostic tests and procedures, and Appendix IV is a list of major medical abbreviations and symbols. Two glossaries, the Glossary of Medical Terms, p. 265, and Glossary of Word Parts, p. 299, are alphabetical listings with definitions of terms and meanings of word parts. Use the appendices and glossaries as references during your study and later as you work in the medical field.

II. BODY CAVITIES

Figure 2-1 shows the five body cavities. A body cavity is a space containing organs. Label Figure 2-1 as you read the following paragraphs.

The **cranial cavity** (1) is located in the head and is surrounded by the skull (CRANI/O means "skull"). The brain and other organs, such as the pituitary gland (an endocrine gland below the brain), are in the cranial cavity.

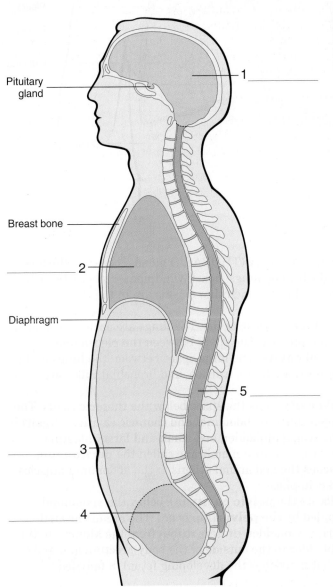

FIGURE 2-1

Body cavities. (Modified from Chabner D-E: *The Language of Medicine,* ed 6, Philadelphia, 2001, WB Saunders.)

FIGURE 2-2

Thoracic cavity.

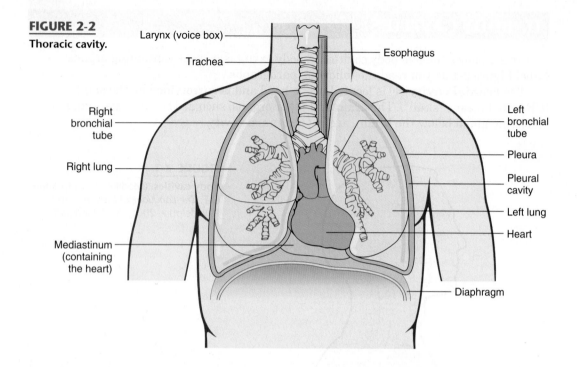

Larynx (voice box)

Trachea

Esophagus

Right bronchial tube

Left bronchial tube

Pleura

Right lung

Pleural cavity

Left lung

Heart

Mediastinum (containing the heart)

Diaphragm

The **thoracic cavity** (2) is the chest cavity (THORAC/O means "chest"), which is surrounded by the breast bone and ribs. The lungs, heart, windpipe (trachea), bronchial tubes (leading from the trachea to the lungs), and other organs are in the thoracic cavity.

Figure 2-2 shows a front view of the thoracic cavity. The lungs are each surrounded by a double membrane known as the **pleura.** The space between the pleura and surrounding each lung is the **pleural cavity.** The large space between the lungs is the **mediastinum.** The heart, esophagus (food tube), trachea, and bronchial tubes are organs within the mediastinum.

In Figure 2-1, the **abdominal cavity** (3) is the space below the thoracic cavity. The **diaphragm** is the muscle that separates the abdominal and thoracic cavities. Organs in the abdomen include the stomach, liver, gallbladder, and small and large intestines.

The organs in the abdomen are covered by a membrane called the **peritoneum** (Figure 2-3). The peritoneum attaches the abdominal organs to the abdominal muscles and surrounds each organ to hold it in place.

Turn back to Figure 2-1 and locate the **pelvic cavity** (4), below the abdominal cavity. The pelvic cavity is surrounded by the **pelvis** (hip bone). The organs located within the pelvic cavity are the urinary bladder, ureters (tubes from the kidneys to the bladder), urethra (tube from the bladder to the outside of the body), rectum and anus, and the uterus (muscular organ that nourishes the developing fetus) in females.

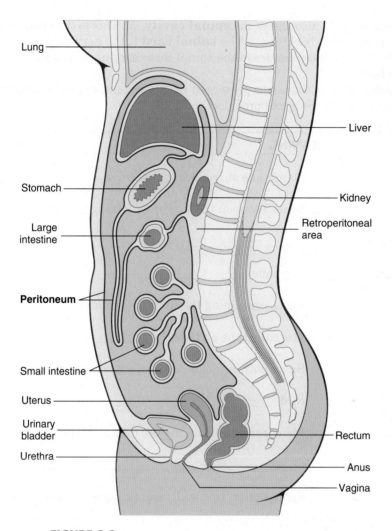

Lung

Liver

Stomach

Kidney

Retroperitoneal
area

Large
intestine

Peritoneum

Small intestine

Uterus

Urinary
bladder

Urethra

Rectum

Anus

Vagina

FIGURE 2-3
The **peritoneum** as it surrounds the organs in the abdomen.

Figure 2-1 on p. 41 also shows the **spinal cavity** (5). This is the space surrounded by the **spinal column** (backbones). The **spinal cord** is the nervous tissue within the spinal cavity. Nerves enter and leave the spinal cord carrying messages to and from all parts of the body.

As a quick review of the terms presented in this section, write the term from the list next to its meaning on the space provided.

TERM	MEANING
Abdominal cavity	1. Membrane surrounding the lungs _____
Cranial cavity	2. Space between the lungs, containing the heart
Diaphragm	_____
Mediastinum	3. Hip bone _____
Pelvic cavity	4. Space containing the liver, gallbladder, and stomach;
Pelvis	also called the abdomen _____
Peritoneum	5. Space within the backbones, containing the spinal
Pleura	cord _____
Spinal cavity	6. Membrane surrounding the organs in the abdomen
Thoracic cavity	_____
	7. Space within the skull, containing the brain
	_____
	8. Space below the abdominal cavity, containing the urinary
	bladder _____
	9. Muscle between the thoracic and abdominal cavities
	_____
	10. Entire chest cavity, containing the lungs, heart, trachea,
	esophagus, and bronchial tubes _____

III. DIVISIONS OF THE BACK

The **spinal column** is a long row of bones from the neck to the tailbone. Each bone in the spinal column is called a **vertebra** (backbone). Two or more bones are **vertebrae.**

A piece of flexible connective tissue, called a **disc** (or **disk**), lies between each backbone. The disk, composed of **cartilage,** is a cushion between the bones. If the disk slips, or moves out of its place, it can press on the nerves that enter or leave the spinal cord and cause pain. Figure 2-4 shows a side view of vertebrae and discs.

The divisions of the spinal column are pictured in Figure 2-5. Label them according to the following list:

DIVISION	BONES	ABBREVIATION
1. **Cervical** (neck) region	7 bones	C1-C7
2. **Thoracic** (chest) region	12 bones	T1-T12
3. **Lumbar** (loin or waist) region	5 bones	L1-L5
4. **Sacral** (sacrum or lower back) region	5 fused bones	S1-S5
5. **Coccygeal** (coccyx or tailbone) region	4 fused bones	

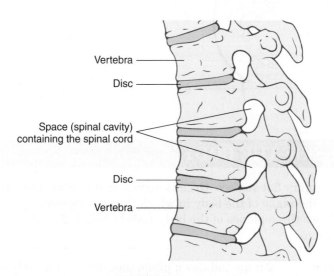

Vertebra

Disc

Space (spinal cavity)
containing the spinal cord

Disc

Vertebra

FIGURE 2-4
Vertebrae and discs.

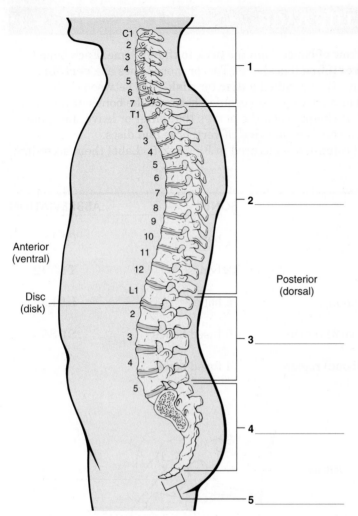

FIGURE 2-5

Divisions of the back. (Modified from Chabner D-E: *The Language of Medicine,* ed 6, Philadelphia, 2001, WB Saunders.)

C1
2
3
4
5
6
7
T1
2
3
4
5
6
7
8
9
10
11
12
L1
2
3
4
5

Anterior (ventral)

Disc (disk)

Posterior (dorsal)

1 _____

2 _____

3 _____

4 _____

5 _____

IV. PLANES OF THE BODY

A plane is an imaginary flat surface. Organs appear in different relationships to each other according to the plane of the body in which they are viewed.

Figure 2-6 shows three planes of the body. Label them *1, 2,* and *3* as you read the following descriptions:

1. **Frontal plane** (sometimes called the coronal plane) — An up-and-down plane that divides the body or an organ into front (**anterior,** or **A**) and back (**posterior,** or **P**) portions. A routine chest x-ray (A/P or P/A) film shows the thoracic cavity in the frontal plane. See Figure 2-7, *A*.

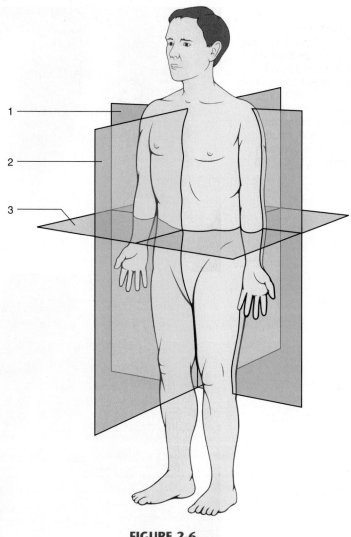

FIGURE 2-6
Planes of the body.

2. **Sagittal (lateral) plane**   A plane that divides the body or an organ into a right and left side. A lateral chest x-ray (see Figure 2-7, *B*, shows the thoracic cavity in the sagittal or lateral plane.

3. **Transverse plane**   A plane that divides the body or an organ into upper and lower portions, as in a **cross-section.** A **CT scan** is an x-ray picture of the body taken in the transverse plane. Figure 2-7, *C*, is a CT scan of the chest.

FIGURE 2-7

X-ray views of the chest. A, Frontal plane. **B,** Sagittal or lateral plane. **C,** Transverse plane. (**A** modified from Black JM, Matassarin-Jacobs E: *Medical-Surgical Nursing: Clinical Management for Continuity of Care,* ed 5, Philadelphia, 1997, WB Saunders. **B** modified from Weir J, Abrahams PH: *An Imaging Atlas of Human Anatomy,* ed 2, London, 2000, Mosby. **C** from Chabner D-E: *The Language of Medicine,* ed 6, Philadelphia, 2001, WB Saunders.)

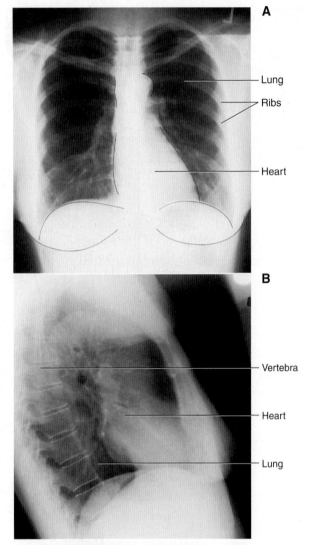

A

— Lung

— Ribs

— Heart

B

— Vertebra

— Heart

— Lung

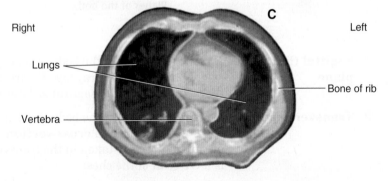

Right

Lungs

Vertebra

C

Left

Bone of rib

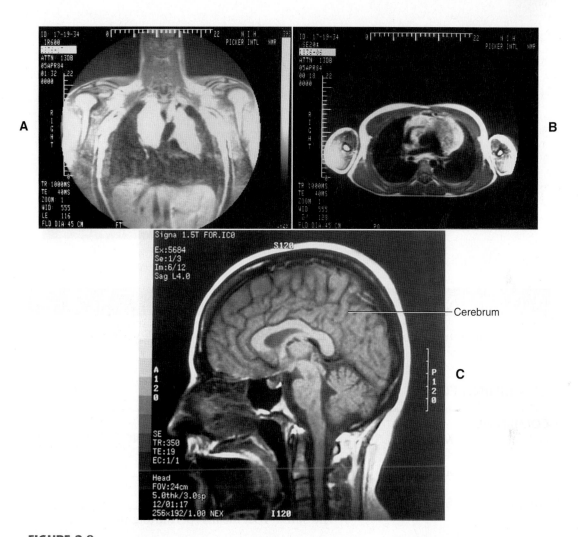

FIGURE 2-8

Magnetic resonance images. A, Frontal view of the upper body. White masses in the chest are tumors.
B, Transverse view of the same patient with a chest mass. **C,** Sagittal (lateral) view of the brain. (**A** and **B**
from Chabner D-E: *The Language of Medicine,* ed 6, Philadelphia, 2001, WB Saunders. **C** modified from Black
JM, Matassarin-Jacobs E: *Medical-Surgical Nursing: Clinical Management for Continuity of Care,* ed 5,
Philadelphia, 1997, WB Saunders.)

Magnetic resonance imaging (MRI) is another technique for producing images of
the body. Instead of x-rays, MRI makes pictures by using magnetic waves. The images
from MRI show organs in all three planes (frontal, sagittal, and transverse) of the body
(Figure 2-8). Figure 2-9 shows a patient undergoing MRI.

FIGURE 2-9

Patient placed within the MRI coils for a head examination. (From Stark DD, Bradley WG: *Magnetic Resonance Imaging,* ed 3, St. Louis, 1999, Mosby.)

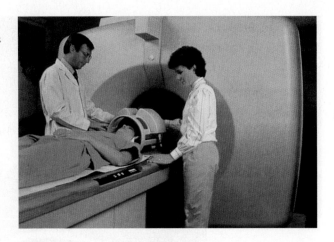

V. TERMINOLOGY

Write the meanings of the medical terms on the line provided. Check your answers with the Glossary at the end of the book or with a medical dictionary.

COMBINING FORMS

COMBINING FORM	MEANING	MEDICAL TERM	MEANING
abdomin/o	abdomen	abdominal	
anter/o	front	anterior _____ The suffix -IOR means "pertaining to."	
bronch/o	bronchial tubes (leading from the windpipe to the lungs)	bronchoscopy	
cervic/o	*neck* of the body or *neck* (cervix) of the uterus	cervical	

You must decide from the context of what you are reading whether *cervical* means "pertaining to the neck of the body" or "pertaining to the cervix" (lower portion of the uterus). Figure 2-10 shows the uterus and the cervix.

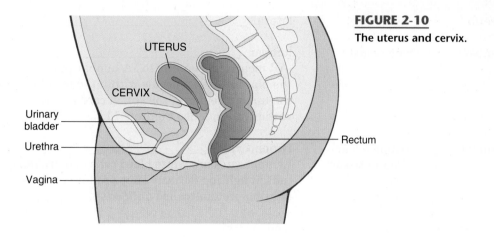

FIGURE 2-10
The uterus and cervix.

| coccyg/o | coccyx, tailbone | coccygeal _____ |
| | | -EAL means "pertaining to." |

| crani/o | skull | craniotomy _____ |

| epitheli/o | skin, surface tissue | epithelial _____ |

The term *epithelial* was first used to describe the surface (EPI- means "upon") of the breast nipple (THELI/O means "nipple"). Currently, it describes the cells on the outer layer (surface) of the skin as well as the lining of the internal organs that lead to the outside of the body.

| esophag/o | esophagus (tube from the throat to the stomach) | esophageal _____ |

| hepat/o | liver | hepatitis _____ |

| lapar/o | abdomen | laparoscopy _____ |

| laryng/o | larynx (voice box) | laryngeal _____ |

The larynx (pronounced **LAR**-inks) is found in the upper part of the trachea.

laryngectomy _____

later/o   side   lateral _____

lumb/o   loin (waist)   lumbar _____
                                    -AR means "pertaining to." A lumbar puncture is
                                    the placement of a needle within the membranes in
                                    the lumbar region of the spinal cord to inject or
                                    withdraw fluid. See Figure 2-11.

lymph/o   lymph (clear   lymphocyte _____
                 fluid in tissue   Lymphocytes are white blood cells and are impor-
                 spaces and   tant in fighting disease. They produce disease-
                 lymph vessels)   fighting proteins called *antibodies*.

mediastin/o   mediastinum   mediastinal _____
                 (space between
                 the lungs)

pelv/o   pelvis (hip bone) pelvic _____

peritone/o   peritoneum   peritoneal _____
                 (membrane sur-
                 rounding the
                 abdomen)

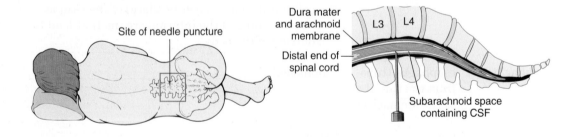

FIGURE 2-11

Lumbar (spinal) puncture. The patient lies laterally, with the knees drawn up to the abdomen and the chin brought down to the chest. This position increases the spaces between the vertebrae. The lumbar puncture needle is inserted between the third and fourth (or fourth and fifth) lumbar vertebrae, and fluid can be injected or withdrawn. The distal end of the spinal cord is where the spinal nerves begin to fan out toward the legs. The lumbar puncture is performed below this area to avoid injury to the spinal cord. (From Chabner D-E: *The Language of Medicine,* ed 6, Philadelphia, 2001, WB Saunders.)

pharyng/o	pharynx (throat)	pharyngeal _____
		The pharynx (pronounced **FAR**-inks) is the common passageway for food from the mouth and air from the nose. See Figure 2-12.
pleur/o	pleura	pleuritis _____
poster/o	back, behind	posterior _____
sacr/o	sacrum (five fused bones in the lower back)	sacral _____
spin/o	spine (backbone)	spinal _____
thorac/o	chest	thoracotomy _____
		thoracic _____
trache/o	trachea (windpipe)	tracheotomy _____
		See Figure 2-13.
vertebr/o	vertebra (backbone)	vertebral _____

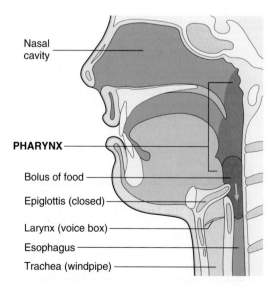

Nasal cavity

PHARYNX

Bolus of food

Epiglottis (closed)

Larynx (voice box)

Esophagus

Trachea (windpipe)

FIGURE 2-12

Pharynx. Notice that the epiglottis (a flap of cartilage) closes over the trachea during swallowing so that the bolus of food travels down the esophagus. (Modified from Chabner D-E: *The Language of Medicine,* ed 6, Philadelphia, 2001, WB Saunders.)

FIGURE 2-13
Tracheotomy.

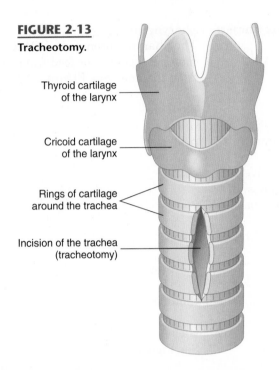

Thyroid cartilage of the larynx

Cricoid cartilage of the larynx

Rings of cartilage around the trachea

Incision of the trachea (tracheotomy)

VI. EXERCISES AND ANSWERS

A. Match the following systems of the body with their functions.

digestive   musculoskeletal   circulatory
respiratory   urinary   endocrine
skin and sense organs   nervous   reproductive

1. Produces urine and sends it out of the body: _____

2. Secretes hormones that are carried by blood to other organs: _____

3. Supports the body and helps it move: _____

4. Takes food into the body and breaks it down: _____

5. Transports food, gases, and other substances through the body: _____

_____

6. Moves air in and out of the body: _____

7. Produces the cells that unite to form a new baby: _____

8. Receives messages from the environment and sends them to the brain: _____

_____

9. Carries electrical messages to and from the brain and spinal cord: _____

_____

◆ **ANSWER KEY**

1. urinary	6. respiratory
2. endocrine	7. reproductive
3. musculoskeletal	8. skin and sense organs
4. digestive	9. nervous
5. circulatory	

B. Use the following terms to complete the chart below. Give the name of the cavity and an organ that is contained within the cavity.

spinal	brain	lungs	urinary bladder
thoracic	pelvic	uterus	spinal cord
stomach	abdominal	cranial	heart

	CAVITY	ORGAN
1. Space contained within the hip bone	_____	_____
2. Space contained within the skull	_____	_____
3. Space contained within the chest	_____	_____
4. Space contained within the abdomen	_____	_____
5. Space contained within the backbones	_____	_____

◆ **ANSWER KEY**
1. pelvic (urinary bladder, uterus)
2. cranial (brain)
3. thoracic (lungs, heart)
4. abdominal (stomach)
5. spinal (spinal cord)

C. Complete the following sentences using the terms listed below.

mediastinum	spinal cord	spinal column
diaphragm	peritoneum	abdomen (abdominal cavity)
disc	vertebra	pleura
pelvis		

1. The hip bone is the _____.

2. The muscle separating the chest and the abdomen is the _____.

3. The membrane surrounding the organs in the abdomen is the _____.

4. The membrane surrounding the lungs is the _____.

5. The space between the lungs in the chest is the _____.

6. The space that contains organs such as the stomach, liver, gallbladder, and

     intestines is the _____.

7. The backbones are the _____.

8. The nerves running down the back form the _____.

9. A single backbone is a _____.

10. A piece of cartilage in between each backbone is a _____.

◆ **ANSWER KEY**

1. pelvis	6. abdomen (abdominal cavity)
2. diaphragm	7. spinal column
3. peritoneum	8. spinal cord
4. pleura	9. vertebra
5. mediastinum	10. disc

D. Name the five divisions of the spinal column from the neck to the tailbone.

1. C ___ ___ ___ ___ ___ ___ ___

2. T ___ ___ ___ ___ ___ ___ ___

3. L ___ ___ ___ ___ ___

4. S __ __ __ __ __

5. C __ __ __ __ __ __ __ __

E. Match the following terms with their meanings below.

transverse plane   CT scan   anterior
frontal plane   sagittal plane   posterior
MRI   cartilage   lateral

1. Pertaining to the back: _____

2. Pertaining to the front: _____

3. A plane that divides the body into an upper and lower part: _____

4. Pertaining to the side: _____

5. A picture of the body using magnetic waves; all three planes of the body can be

   viewed: _____

6. A plane that divides the body into right and left parts: _____

7. Flexible connective tissue found between bones at joints: _____

8. A plane that divides the body into front and back parts: _____

9. Series of x-ray pictures taken in cross-section: _____

F. Give meanings for the following terms.

1. craniotomy _____

2. abdominal _____

3. pelvic _____

4. thoracic _____

5. mediastinal _____

6. epithelial _____

7. tracheotomy _____

8. peritoneal _____

9. hepatitis _____

10. cervical _____

11. lymphocyte _____

12. lateral _____

13. bronchoscopy _____

14. diaphragm _____

15. pleura _____

12. pertaining to the side
13. visual examination of the bronchial tubes
14. muscle separating the abdomen from the chest
15. membrane surrounding the lungs

G. Match the following terms with their meanings below.

pleuritis	pharyngeal	laryngeal	esophageal
epithelial	coccygeal	thoracotomy	lumbar
vertebral	laparoscopy	laparotomy	sacral

1. Pertaining to the loin (waist) region directly under the thoracic vertebrae: _____

_____

2. Pertaining to skin or surface cells: _____

3. Incision of the abdomen: _____

4. Pertaining to the food tube: _____

5. Pertaining to the voice box: _____

6. Inflammation of the membrane surrounding the lungs: _____

7. Pertaining to the throat: _____

8. Pertaining to the sacrum: _____

9. Incision of the chest: _____

10. Pertaining to the tailbone: _____

11. Visual examination of the abdomen: _____

12. Pertaining to backbones: _____

◆ **ANSWER KEY**

1. lumbar
2. epithelial
3. laparotomy
4. esophageal
5. laryngeal
6. pleuritis

7. pharyngeal
8. sacral
9. thoracotomy
10. coccygeal
11. laparoscopy
12. vertebral

H. Circle the term that best completes the meaning of the sentences in the following medical vignettes.

1. After her car accident, Cathy had severe neck pain. An MRI revealed a protruding **(diaphragm, disc, uterus)** at the C7 **(coccyx, ovary, vertebra)**. The doctor asked her to wear a **(sacral, cervical, cranial)** collar for several weeks.

2. Mr. Sellar was a heavy smoker all his adult life. He began coughing and losing weight and became very lethargic (tired). His physician suspected a tumor of the **(musculoskeletal, urinary, respiratory)** system. A chest CT demonstrated a **(mediastinal, pharyngeal, spinal)** mass. Dr. Baker performed **(laparoscopy, craniotomy, bronchoscopy)** to biopsy the lesion.

3. Grace had never seen a gynecologist. She had pain in her **(cranial, pelvic, thoracic)** cavity and increasing **(abdominal, vertebral, laryngeal)** girth or size. Dr. Hawk suspected a(an) **(esophageal, ovarian, mediastinal)** tumor, after palpating (examining by touch) a mass.

4. Mr. Cruise worked in the shipyards for several years during World War II. Now, many years later, his doctor encouraged him to stop smoking because of a recently discovered link between asbestos, smoking, and the occurrence of mesothelioma (malignant tumor of cells found in the membrane surrounding the lungs). On a routine chest x-ray, there had been thickening of the **(esophagus, pleura, trachea)** on both sides of Mr. Cruise's **(abdominal, spinal, thoracic)** cavity.

5. When Kelly complained of headaches, together with nausea, disturbances of vision, loss of coordination in her movements, weakness, and stiffness on one side of her body, Dr. Brown suspected a tumor of the central **(circulatory, digestive, nervous)** system. Treatment involved a **(thoracotomy, craniotomy, laryngectomy)** to remove the mass in her brain.

6. Mr. Jones experienced increasing weakness and loss of movement in his left arm and left leg. He saw his family doctor, who immediately referred him to a **(neurologist, cardiologist, rheumatologist)**. The specialist examined him and sent him to **(pathology, hematology, radiology)** for x-ray imaging. (His results are shown in Figure 2-14.) This procedure produced a(an) **(MRI, CT scan, A/P film)**. The imaging clearly showed a large white region in the brain, indicating an area of dead tissue. Mr. Jones' doctor informed him that he had had a stroke, which is also known as a **(pituitary gland tumor, myocardial infarction, CVA or cerebrovascular accident)**.

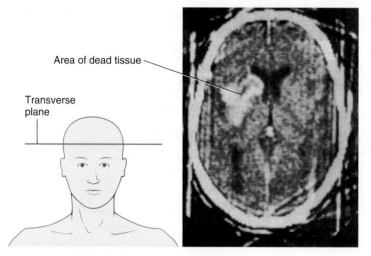

FIGURE 2-14
Cross-sectional x-ray image of Mr. Smith's head.

Area of dead tissue

Transverse plane

◆ **ANSWER KEY**
1. disc, vertebra, cervical
2. respiratory, mediastinal, bronchoscopy
3. pelvic, abdominal, ovarian
4. pleura, thoracic
5. nervous, craniotomy
6. neurologist, radiology, CT scan, CVA or cerebrovascular accident

VII. REVIEW

Write the meanings of the following combining forms and suffixes in the space provided. Be sure to check your answers with the answer key at the end of each list.

COMBINING FORMS

COMBINING FORM	MEANING	COMBINING FORM	MEANING
1. abdomin/o	_____	4. cervic/o	_____
2. anter/o	_____	5. coccygo/o	_____
3. bronch/o	_____	6. crani/o	_____

7. epitheli/o _____

8. esophag/o _____

9. hepat/o _____

10. lapar/o _____

11. laryng/o _____

12. later/o _____

13. lumb/o _____

14. lymph/o _____

15. mediastin/o _____

16. pelv/o _____

17. peritone/o _____

18. pharyng/o _____

19. pleur/o _____

20. poster/o _____

21. sacr/o _____

22. spin/o _____

23. thorac/o _____

24. trache/o _____

25. vertebr/o _____

SUFFIXES

SUFFIX	MEANING	SUFFIX	MEANING
1. -ac	_____	6. -ic	_____
2. -al	_____	8. -itis	_____
3. -ar	_____	9. -logy	_____
4. -cyte	_____	10. -oma	_____
5. -eal	_____	11. -scopy	_____
6. -ectomy	_____	12. -tomy	_____

COMBINING FORMS

◆ **ANSWER KEY**

1. abdomen
2. front
3. bronchial tubes
4. neck
5. tailbone
6. skull
7. skin
8. esophagus
9. liver
10. abdomen

11. voice box
12. side
13. loin, waist region
14. lymph
15. mediastinum
16. hip bone
17. peritoneum
18. throat
19. pleura
20. back, behind
21. sacrum
22. backbone
23. chest
24. windpipe
25. backbone

SUFFIXES

1. pertaining to
2. pertaining to
3. pertaining to
4. cell
5. pertaining to
6. removal, excision, resection
7. pertaining to
8. inflammation
9. study of
10. tumor, mass
11. process of viewing
12. incision, to cut into

VIII. PRONUNCIATION OF TERMS

The terms that you have learned in this chapter are presented here with their pronunciations. The capitalized letters in boldface represent the accented syllable. Pronounce each word out loud, then write the meaning in the space provided.

TERM	PRONUNCIATION	MEANING
abdomen	**AB**-do-men	
abdominal cavity	ab-**DOM**-in-al **KAV**-i-te	
anterior	an-**TE**-re-or	
bronchial tubes	**BRONG**-ke-al tubes	
bronchoscopy	bron-**KOS**-ko-pe	
cartilage	**KAR**-tih-lij	
cervical	**SER**-vi-kal	
circulatory system	**SER**-ku-lah-tor-e **SIS**-tem	

coccygeal   kok-sih-**JE**-al _____

coccyx   **KOK**-siks _____

cranial cavity   **KRA**-ne-al **KAV**-ih-te _____

craniotomy   kra-ne-**OT**-o-me _____

diaphragm   **DI**-ah-fram _____

digestive system   di-**JES**-tiv **SIS**-tem _____

disc (disk)   disk _____

endocrine system   **EN**-do-krin **SIS**-tem _____

epithelial   ep-ih-**THE**-le-al _____

esophageal   eh-sof-ah-**JE**-al _____

esophagus   eh-**SOF**-ah-gus _____

female reproductive   **FE**-mal re-pro-**DUK**-tiv **SIS**-tem _____
system

frontal plane   **FRUN**-tal plan _____

hepatitis   hep-ah-**TI**-tis _____

laparoscopy   lap-ah-**ROS**-ko-pe _____

laparotomy   lap-ah-**ROT**-o-me _____

laryngeal   lah-**RIN**-je-al or lah-rin-**JE**-al _____

laryngectomy   lah-rin-**JEK**-to-me _____

larynx   **LAR**-inks _____

lateral   **LAT**-er-al _____

lumbar   **LUM**-bar _____

lymphocyte   **LIMF**-o-site _____

mediastinal	me-de-as-**TI**-nal _____
mediastinum	me-de-ahs-**TI**-num _____
musculoskeletal system	mus-ku-lo-**SKEL**-e-tal **SIS**-tem _____
nervous system	**NER**-vus **SIS**-tem _____
ovary	**O**-vah-re _____
pelvic cavity	**PEL**-vik **KAV**-ih-te _____
pelvis	**PEL**-vis _____
peritoneal	per-ih-to-**NE**-al _____
peritoneum	per-ih-to-**NE**-um _____
pharyngeal	fah-**RIN**-je-al or fah-rin-**JE**-al _____
pharynx	**FAR**-inks _____
pituitary gland	pih-**TU**-ih-tah-re gland _____
pleura	**PLOO**-rah _____
pleuritis	ploo-**RI**-tis _____
posterior	pos-**TER**-e-or _____
respiratory system	**RES**-pir-ah-tor-e **SIS**-tem _____
sacral	**SA**-kral _____
sacrum	**SA**-krum _____
sagittal plane	**SAJ**-ih-tal plan _____
spinal cavity	**SPI**-nal **KAV**-ih-te _____
spinal column	**SPI**-nal **KOL**-um _____
spinal cord	**SPI**-nal kord _____

thoracic cavity	tho-**RAS**-ik **KAV**-ih-te _____
thoracotomy	tho-rah-**KOT**-o-me _____
trachea	**TRAY**-ke-ah _____
tracheotomy	tray-ke-**OT**-o-me _____
transverse plane	trans-**VERS** plan _____
ureter	**YOOR**-eh-ter or u-**RE**-ter _____
urethra	u-**RE**-thrah _____
urinary system	**UR**-in-er-e **SIS**-tem _____
uterus	**U**-ter-us _____
vertebra	**VER**-teh-brah _____
vertebrae	**VER**-teh-bray _____
vertebral	**VER**-teh-bral _____

IX. PRACTICAL APPLICATIONS

The following are descriptions of surgical procedures. Can you identify the procedure from its description below? Your choices are:

laparoscopy   craniotomy   tracheotomy
laparotomy   bronchoscopy   thoracotomy
laryngectomy

1. A skin incision is made, and muscle is stripped away from the skull. Four or five burr (bur) holes are drilled into the skull. The bone between the holes is cut using a craniotome (bone saw). The bone flap is turned down or completely removed. After the bone flap is secured, the membrane surrounding the brain is incised and the brain is exposed. This procedure is called a _____.

2. A major surgical incision is made into the chest for diagnostic or therapeutic purposes. One type of incision is a medial sternotomy (the sternum is the breast bone). A straight incision is made from the upper part of the sternum (suprasternal notch) to the lower end of the sternum (xiphoid process). The sternum must be cut with an electric or air-driven saw. The procedure is done to perform a biopsy or to locate sources of bleeding or injury. It is often performed to remove all or a portion of the lung. This procedure is known

as a _____.

3. A needle is inserted below the umbilicus (navel) to infuse carbon dioxide (a gas) into the abdomen. This distends (expands) the abdomen and permits better visualization of the organs. A trocar (sharp-pointed instrument used to puncture the wall of a body cavity) within a cannula (tube) is inserted into an incision under the umbilicus. After it is in place in the abdominal cavity, the trocar is removed and an endoscope is inserted through the cannula. The surgeon can thus visualize the abdominopelvic cavity and reproductive organs. This procedure is

known as a _____.

4. A flexible, fiberoptic endoscope is inserted through the mouth, nose, throat, and trachea to assess the tracheobronchial tree for tumors and obstructions, to perform biopsies, and to remove secretions and foreign bodies. This procedure is

called a _____.

◆ **ANSWER KEY**   1. craniotomy   3. laparoscopy
               2. thoracotomy   4. bronchoscopy

SUFFIXES

CHAPTER SECTIONS

CHAPTER OBJECTIVES

- To identify and define useful diagnostic and procedural suffixes
- To analyze, spell, and pronounce medical terms that contain diagnostic and procedural suffixes

I. INTRODUCTION

This chapter reviews the suffixes that you have learned in the first two chapters and also introduces new suffixes and medical terms. The combining forms used in the chapter are listed below in Section II. Refer to this list as you write the meanings of the terms in Section III. Be faithful about completing the Exercises in Section IV, and remember to check your answers! These exercises will help you spell terms correctly and understand their meanings. Test yourself by completing the Review in Section V and Pronunciation of Terms in Section VI.

II. COMBINING FORMS

COMBINING FORM	MEANING
aden/o	gland
amni/o	amnion (sac of fluid surrounding the embryo)
angi/o	vessel (usually a blood vessel)
arteri/o	artery
arthr/o	joint
ather/o	plaque (a yellow, fatty material)
axill/o	armpit (underarm)
bronch/o	bronchial tubes
bronchi/o	bronchial tubes
carcin/o	cancerous
cardi/o	heart
chem/o	drug (or chemical)
cholecyst/o	gallbladder
chron/o	time
col/o	colon (large intestine or bowel)
crani/o	skull
cry/o	cold
cyst/o	urinary bladder; also a sac of fluid or cyst
electr/o	electricity
encephal/o	brain
erythr/o	red
esophag/o	esophagus (tube leading from the throat to the stomach)
hem/o	blood
hemat/o	blood
hepat/o	liver
hyster/o	uterus
inguin/o	groin (the depression between the thigh and the trunk of the body)

isch/o	to hold back
lapar/o	abdomen (abdominal wall)
laryng/o	voice box (larynx)
leuk/o	white
mamm/o	breast (use with -ARY, -GRAPHY, -GRAM, and -PLASTY)
mast/o	breast (use with -ECTOMY and -ITIS)
men/o	menses (menstruation); month
mening/o	meninges (membranes around the brain and spinal cord)
my/o	muscle
myel/o	spinal cord (nervous tissue connected to the brain and located within the spinal column or backbone); in other terms, MYEL/O- means bone marrow (the soft, inner part of bones, where blood cells are made)
necr/o	death (of cells)
nephr/o	kidney (use with all suffixes, except -AL and -GRAM; use REN/O with -AL and -GRAM)
neur/o	nerve
oophor/o	ovary
oste/o	bone
ot/o	ear
pelv/o	pelvic bone (hip bone)
peritone/o	peritoneum (membrane surrounding the organs in the abdominal cavity)
phleb/o	vein
pneumon/o	lung
pulmon/o	lung
radi/o	x-rays
ren/o	kidney (use with -AL and -GRAM)
rhin/o	nose
salping/o	fallopian (uterine) tubes
sarc/o	flesh
septic/o	pertaining to infection
thorac/o	chest
tonsill/o	tonsils
trache/o	windpipe; trachea
ur/o	urine or urea (waste material); urinary tract
vascul/o	blood vessel

III. SUFFIXES AND TERMINOLOGY

Suffixes are divided into two groups, those that describe **diagnoses** and those that describe **procedures**.

DIAGNOSTIC SUFFIXES

These suffixes describe disease conditions or their symptoms. Use the list of combining forms in the previous section to write the meaning of each term. You will find it helpful to check the meanings of the terms with the glossary at the end of book or with a medical dictionary.

NOUN SUFFIX	MEANING	TERMINOLOGY	MEANING
-algia	pain	arthralgia _____	
		otalgia _____	
		myalgia _____	
		neuralgia _____	
-emia	blood condition	leukemia _____ Increase in numbers of leukocytes; cells are malignant (cancerous).	
		septicemia _____	
		ischemia _____ Figure 3-1 illustrates ischemia of heart muscle caused by blockage of a coronary (heart) artery.	
		uremia _____ Uremia occurs when the kidneys fail to function and urea (waste material) accumulates in the blood.	
-ia	condition, disease	pneumonia _____ The lung is inflamed, and fluid or material collects in the air sacs of the lung.	
-itis	inflammation	bronchitis _____ See Figure 3-2.	
		esophagitis _____	
		laryngitis _____	

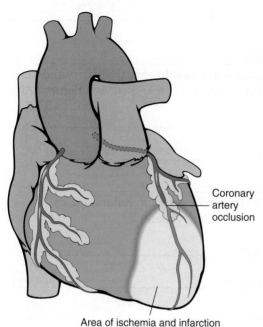

FIGURE 3-1

Ischemia of heart muscle. Blood is held back from an area of heart muscle by an occlusion (blockage) of a coronary (heart) artery. The muscle then loses its supply of oxygen and food and, if the condition persists, dies. The death of the heart muscle is known as a heart attack (myocardial infarction). (From Chabner D-E: *The Language of Medicine,* ed 6, Philadelphia, 2001, WB Saunders.)

Coronary artery occlusion

Area of ischemia and infarction

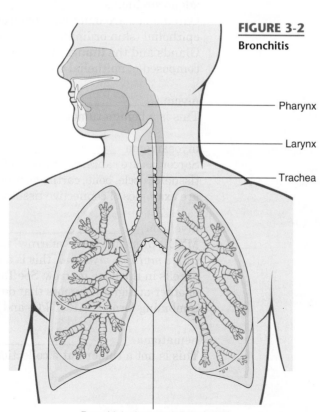

FIGURE 3-2
Bronchitis

Pharynx

Larynx

Trachea

Bronchial tubes are inflamed with hypersecretion of mucus

meningitis _____

The meninges are membranes that surround and protect the brain and spinal cord. See Figure 3-3.

cystitis _____

phlebitis _____

colitis _____

Table 3-1 lists other common inflammatory conditions with their meanings.

-megaly   enlargement   cardiomegaly _____

hepatomegaly _____

-oma   tumor, mass   adenoma _____

This is a benign (non-cancerous) tumor.

adenocarcinoma _____

Carcinomas are malignant (cancerous) tumors of epithelial (skin or lining) tissue in the body. Glands and the linings of internal organs are composed of epithelial tissue.

myoma _____

This is a benign tumor.

myosarcoma _____

Sarcomas are cancerous tumors of connective (flesh) tissue. Muscle, bone, cartilage, fibrous tissue, and fat are examples of connective tissues. See Table 3-2.

myeloma _____

MYEL/O- means "bone marrow" in this term. Also called *multiple myeloma,* this is a malignant tumor of cells in the bone marrow. See Table 3-3 for names of other malignant tumors that do not contain the combining forms, CARCIN/O- and SARC/O-.

hematoma _____

This is not a tumor but a collection of fluid (blood).

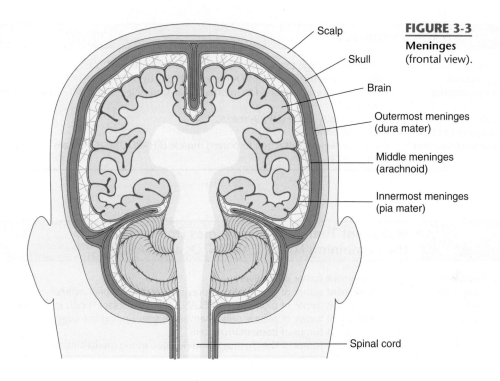

FIGURE 3-3

Meninges (frontal view).

Scalp

Skull

Brain

Outermost meninges (dura mater)

Middle meninges (arachnoid)

Innermost meninges (pia mater)

Spinal cord

TABLE 3-1	Inflammations

appendicitis	Inflammation of the appendix (hangs from the colon in the lower right abdomen)
bursitis	Inflammation of a small sac of fluid (bursa) near a joint
cellulitis	Inflammation of soft tissue under the skin
dermatitis	Inflammation of the skin
endocarditis	Inflammation of the inner lining of the heart (endocardium)
epiglottitis	Inflammation of the epiglottis (cartilage at the upper part of the windpipe)
gastritis	Inflammation of the stomach
hepatitis	Inflammation of the liver
myositis	Inflammation of muscle (MYOS/O- means "muscle.")
nephritis	Inflammation of the kidney
osteomyelitis	Inflammation of bone and bone marrow
otitis	Inflammation of the ear
pharyngitis	Inflammation of the throat
thrombophlebitis	Inflammation of a vein with formation of clots

TABLE 3-2 ◇ **Sarcomas**	
chondrosarcoma	Cancer of cartilage tissue (CHONDR/O- means "cartilage.")
fibrosarcoma	Cancer of fibrous tissue (FIBR/O- means "fibrous tissue.")
leiomyosarcoma	Cancer of visceral (attached to internal organs) muscle (LEIOMY/O- means "visceral muscle")
liposarcoma	Cancer of fatty tissue (LIP/O- means "fat.")
osteogenic sarcoma	Cancer of bone
rhabdomyosarcoma	Cancer of skeletal (attached to bones) muscle (RHABDOMY/O- means "skeletal muscle.")

TABLE 3-3 ◇ **Malignant Tumors Whose Names Do Not Contain the Combining Forms CARCIN/O- and SARC/O-**	
hepatoma	Malignant tumor of the liver
lymphoma	Malignant tumor of lymph nodes (previously called *lymphosarcoma*)
melanoma	Malignant tumor of pigmented (MELAN/O- means "black") cells in the skin
mesothelioma	Malignant tumor of pleural cells (membrane surrounding the lungs)
multiple myeloma	Malignant tumor of bone marrow cells
thymoma	Malignant tumor of the thymus gland (located in the mediastinum)

-osis	condition, abnormal condition	nephrosis _____
		necrosis _____
		erythrocytosis _____ When -OSIS is used with blood cell words, it means "a slight increase in numbers of cells."
		leukocytosis _____ This condition occurs as a normal response to infection.
-pathy	disease condition	encephalopathy _____ Pronunciation is en-sef-ah-**LOP**-ah-the.
		cardiomyopathy _____ Pronunciation is kar-de-o-mi-**OP**-ah-the.
		nephropathy _____ Pronunciation is neh-**FROP**-ah-the. Table 3-4 lists other disease conditions.

TABLE 3-4	Disease Conditions (-PATHIES)
adrenopathy	Disease condition of the adrenal glands
hepatopathy	Disease condition of the liver
lymphadenopathy	Disease condition of the lymph nodes (previously called *glands*)
myopathy	Disease condition of muscles
neuropathy	Disease condition of nerves
osteopathy	Disease condition of bones
retinopathy	Disease condition of the retina of the eye

-rrhea   flow, discharge   rhinorrhea _____

menorrhea _____
Normal menstrual flow.

-rrhage or bursting forth of hemorrhage _____
-rrhagia   blood

menorrhagia _____
Excessive bleeding during menstruation.

-sclerosis   hardening   arteriosclerosis _____
Atherosclerosis is the most common type of
arteriosclerosis. A fatty plaque (atheroma) collects
on the lining of arteries. See Figure 3-4.

-uria   condition of urine hematuria _____
Bleeding into the urinary tract can cause this
condition.

All the following **adjective suffixes** mean "pertaining to" and *describe* a part of the
body, process, or condition.

-al or -eal pertaining to   peritoneal _____

inguinal _____

renal _____

esophageal _____

FIGURE 3-4

Atherosclerosis (type of arteriosclerosis). A fatty (cholesterol) material collects in an artery, narrowing it and eventually blocking the flow of blood.

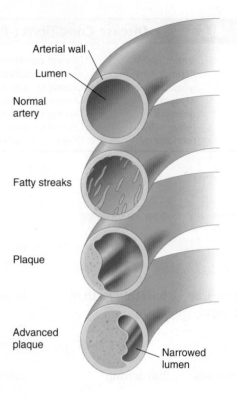

Arterial wall

Lumen

Normal artery

Fatty streaks

Plaque

Advanced plaque

Narrowed lumen

myocardial _____
A heart attack is also called a *myocardial infarction* (MI). An infarction is an area of dead tissue caused by ischemia (when blood supply is held back from a part of the body).

-ar   pertaining to   vascular _____
A *cerebrovascular accident* (CVA) is a stroke.

-ary   pertaining to   axillary _____

mammary _____

pulmonary _____

-ic   pertaining to   chronic _____
Chronic conditions occur over a long period of time, as opposed to *acute* conditions, which are sharp, sudden, and brief.

pelvic _____

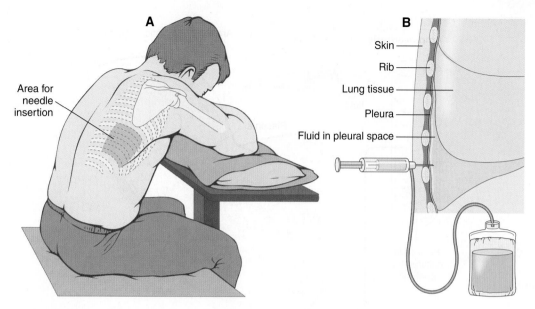

FIGURE 3-5

Technique of thoracentesis. A, The patient is sitting in the correct position for the procedure. **B,** The needle is advanced, and the fluid (pleural effusion) is drained.

PROCEDURAL SUFFIXES

The following suffixes describe *procedures* used in patient care.

SUFFIX	MEANING	TERMINOLOGY	MEANING
-centesis	surgical puncture to remove fluid	thoracentesis _____ The term is a shortened form of thoracocentesis. See Figure 3-5.	
		amniocentesis _____ See Figure 3-6.	
		arthrocentesis _____	
-ectomy	removal, resection, excision	tonsillectomy _____ Tonsils and adenoids are *lymph tissue* in the pharynx (throat). Lymph is composed of white blood cells that fight infection. See Figure 3-7.	

FIGURE 3-6

Amniocentesis.

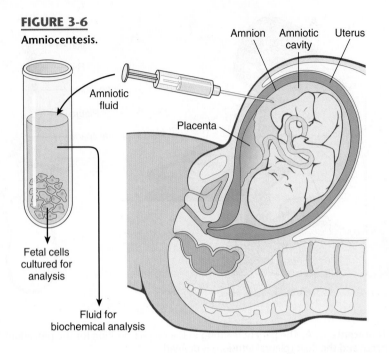

FIGURE 3-7

Tonsils and adenoids. A tonsillectomy and adenoidectomy (T&A) is removal of the tonsils and adenoids.

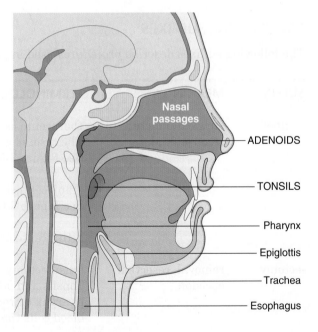

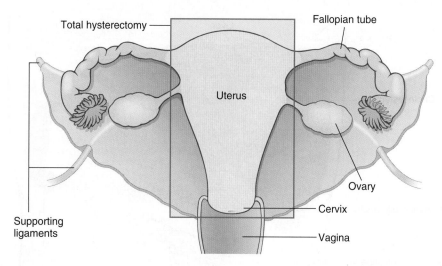

FIGURE 3-8

Total hysterectomy. In a total abdominal hysterectomy (TAH), the uterus is removed through the abdomen. A TAH-BSO is a total abdominal hysterectomy with bilateral salpingectomy and oophorectomy.

hysterectomy _____
In a *total* hysterectomy, the whole uterus, including the cervix, is removed. If a portion of the uterus is not removed, the procedure is termed a *partial* or *subtotal* hysterectomy. See Figure 3-8.

oophorectomy _____

salpingectomy _____

cholecystectomy _____
See Figure 3-9.

mastectomy _____
Table 3-5 lists additional resection procedures.

-gram   record   myelogram _____
MYEL/O- means "spinal cord" in this term. A contrast material is injected into the membranes around the spinal cord (by *lumbar puncture*), and then x-ray pictures are taken of the spinal cord. This procedure is performed less frequently now that MRI is available.

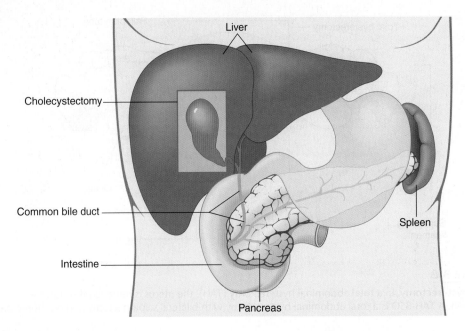

FIGURE 3-9

Cholecystectomy. The liver is lifted up to show the gallbladder underneath. The pancreas is a long, thin gland located behind and to the left of the stomach, toward the spleen. The common bile duct carries bile from the liver and gallbladder to the intestine.

TABLE 3-5 ◆ Resections	
adenectomy	Excision of a gland
adenoidectomy	Excision of the adenoids
appendectomy	Excision of the appendix
colectomy	Excision of the colon
gastrectomy	Excision of the stomach
laminectomy	Excision of a piece of backbone (lamina) to relieve pressure on nerves from a (herniating) disc
myomectomy	Excision of a muscle tumor (commonly a fibroid of the uterus)
pneumonectomy	Excision of lung tissue; total pneumonectomy (an entire lung), or lobectomy (a single lobe)
splenectomy	Excision of the spleen

		mammogram _____ See Figure 3-10.
-graphy	process of recording	electroencephalography _____
		mammography _____ See Figure 3-11.

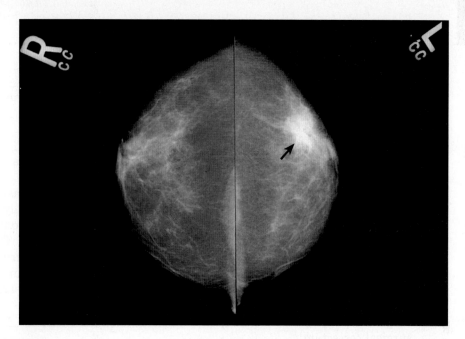

FIGURE 3-10

Mammograms of a 63-year-old woman. The right breast is normal, and the left breast contains a breast cancer *(arrow)*. (From Ballinger PW, Frank ED: *Merrill's Atlas of Radiographic Positions and Radiographic Procedures,* ed 9, vol 2, St Louis, 1999, Mosby.)

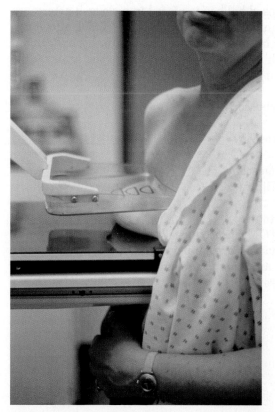

FIGURE 3-11

Mammography. The breast is compressed and x-rays images *(top to bottom and lateral)* are taken. (Courtesy Dr. Elizabeth Chabner Thompson.)

angiography _____
Arteriography, phlebography (veins), and lymphangiography are examples of angiography.

-lysis   separation, break-   dialysis _____
            down, destruction   *Hemodialysis* is the removal of blood and its
passage through (DIA- means "through or
complete") a kidney machine to filter out waste
materials, such as *urea*. Another form of dialysis is
peritoneal dialysis. A special fluid is put into the
peritoneum through a tube in the abdomen. The
wastes seep into the fluid from the blood during a
period of time. The fluid and wastes are then
drained from the peritoneum. See Figure 3-12.

-plasty   surgical repair, or   mammoplasty _____
            surgical correction

rhinoplasty _____

angioplasty _____
Balloon angioplasty is performed on the coronary
arteries that surround the heart. A wire with a
collapsed balloon is placed in a clogged artery.
Opening the balloon widens the vessel, allowing
more blood to flow through. Currently, a **stent**
(mesh rodlike device) is placed in the artery to
hold it open. See Figure 3-13.

-scopy   process of visual   bronchoscopy _____
            examination

laparoscopy _____

laryngoscopy _____
See Figure 3-14.

-stomy   opening   colostomy _____
A -STOMY procedure is the creation of a
permanent or semipermanent opening (stoma)
from an organ to the outside of the body. See
Figure 3-15.

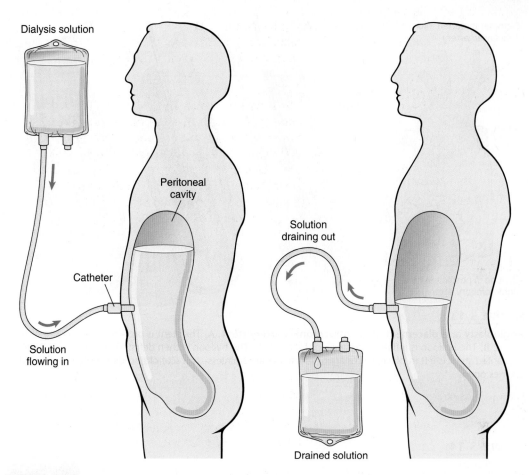

FIGURE 3-12

Peritoneal dialysis. This procedure (or the alternative method of hemodialysis) is necessary when the kidneys are not functioning to remove waste materials (such as urea) from the blood. Without dialysis or kidney transplantation, uremia can result. (From Chabner D-E: *The Language of Medicine,* ed 6, Philadelphia, 2001, WB Saunders.)

		tracheostomy _____
		See Figure 3-16.
-therapy	treatment	radiotherapy _____
		chemotherapy _____

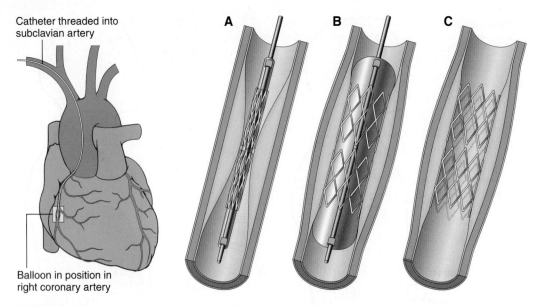

Catheter threaded into
subclavian artery

A **B** **C**

Balloon in position in
right coronary artery

FIGURE 3-13

Angioplasty and placement of an intracoronary artery stent. A, The stent is positioned at the site of the lesion. **B,** The balloon is inflated, expanding the stent. **C,** The balloon is then deflated and removed, and the implanted stent is left in place. Coronary artery stents are stainless-steel scaffolding devices that help hold arteries open.

FIGURE 3-14

Laryngoscopy.

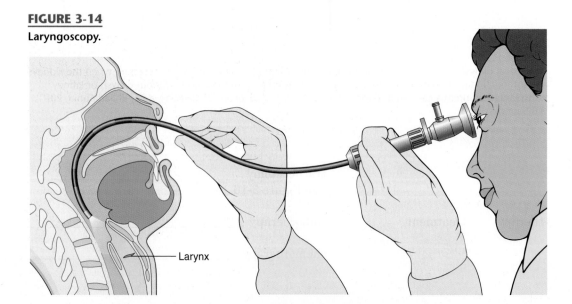

Larynx

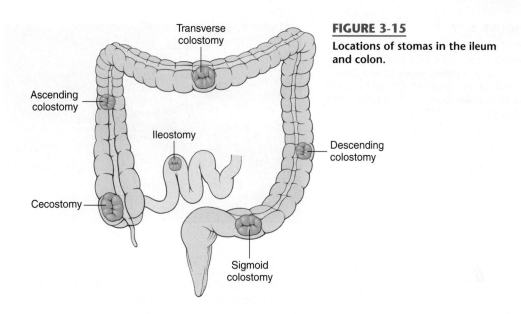

FIGURE 3-15

Locations of stomas in the ileum and colon.

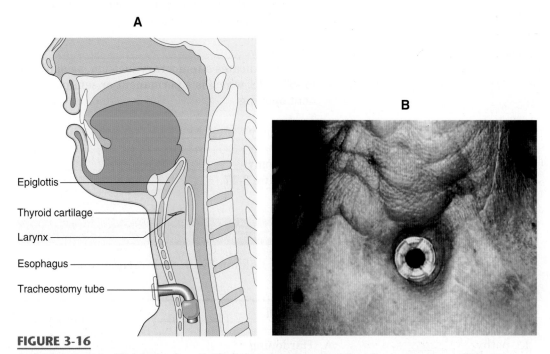

FIGURE 3-16

A, Tracheostomy, with tube in place. **B, Healed tracheostomy incision** after laryngectomy. (**B** from Black JM, Matassarin-Jacobs E: *Medical-Surgical Nursing: Clinical Management for Continuity of Care,* ed 5, Philadelphia, 1997, WB Saunders.)

FIGURE 3-17

Phlebotomy. After entering a vein with a needle through the skin, the plunger of the syringe is pulled slowly to withdraw blood. (From Zakus SM: *Clinical Procedure for Medical Assistants,* ed 3, St Louis, 1995, Mosby.)

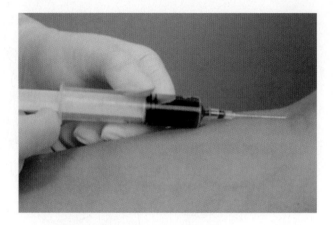

cryotherapy _____
Cryoextraction is the application of extremely low temperature for the removal of a cataractous lens of the eye. Cryocautery is the burning (cauterization) of tissue by the application of liquid nitrogen, carbon dioxide snow, or an instrument that destroys tissue by freezing.

-tomy   incision, to cut into

craniotomy _____
-TOMY indicates a temporary incision, as opposed to -STOMY, which is a permanent or semipermanent opening.

laparotomy _____

phlebotomy _____
See Figure 3-17.

IV. EXERCISES AND ANSWERS

A. Match the following diagnostic suffixes in Column I with their meanings in Column II.

COLUMN I		COLUMN II
1. -pathy	____	A. Hardening
2. -rrhea	____	B. Discharge, flow

3. -algia	____	C. Inflammation
4. -oma	____	D. Blood condition
5. -itis	____	E. Pain
6. -rrhagia	____	F. Enlargement
7. -sclerosis	____	G. Disease condition
8. -osis	____	H. Tumor, mass
9. -emia	____	I. Bursting forth of blood
10. -megaly	____	J. Abnormal condition

◆ **ANSWER KEY**
1. G	2. B	3. E	4. H	5. C
6. I	7. A	8. J	9. D	10. F

B. Match the following procedural suffixes in Column I with their meanings in Column II.

COLUMN I		COLUMN II
1. -tomy	____	A. Removal, resection, excision
2. -scopy	____	B. Visual examination
3. -therapy	____	C. Process of recording
4. -stomy	____	D. Opening
5. -lysis	____	E. Record
6. -centesis	____	F. Separation, breakdown, destruction
7. -plasty	____	G. Treatment
8. -graphy	____	H. Surgical repair
9. -ectomy	____	I. Incision, to cut into
10. -gram	____	J. Surgical puncture to remove fluid

C. Select from the following terms to complete the sentences below:

myalgia   angioplasty   hematuria
septicemia   rhinorrhea   leukemia
thoracentesis   menorrhagia   arteriosclerosis
laryngitis   esophagitis   ischemia

1. Surgical puncture to remove fluid from the chest is _____

2. Surgical repair of a blood vessel is _____

3. Muscle pain is _____

4. Inflammation of the tube leading from the throat to the stomach is _____

   _____

5. Holding back blood from an organ or depriving it of blood supply is _____

   _____

6. Discharge of mucus from the nose is _____

7. Blood in the urine is _____

8. A malignant condition of abnormal increase in white blood cells is _____

   _____

9. Hardening of arteries is _____

10. Excessive discharge of blood during menstruation is _____

11. Inflammation of the voice box is known as _____

12. A blood infection is _____

◆ **ANSWER KEY**

1. thoracentesis
2. angioplasty
3. myalgia
4. esophagitis
5. ischemia
6. rhinorrhea
7. hematuria
8. leukemia
9. arteriosclerosis
10. menorrhagia
11. laryngitis
12. septicemia

D. Underline the suffix and give meanings for the following terms:

1. bronchitis _____

2. encephalopathy _____

3. pelvic _____

4. carcinoma _____

5. chronic _____

6. otalgia _____

7. inguinal _____

8. mastectomy _____

9. colostomy _____

10. leukocytosis _____

11. cardiomegaly _____

12. hematuria _____

13. uremia _____

14. necrosis _____

15. cryotherapy _____

◆ **ANSWER KEY**
1. bronchitis—inflammation of bronchial tubes
2. encephalopathy—disease of the brain
3. pelvic—pertaining to the hip bone
4. carcinoma—cancerous tumor (of epithelial or skin tissue)
5. chronic—pertaining to occurring over a long period of time
6. otalgia—pain in the ear (earache)
7. inguinal—pertaining to the groin
8. mastectomy—removal of a breast
9. colostomy—opening of the colon to the outside of the body
10. leukocytosis—abnormal condition (slight increase) of white blood cells
11. cardiomegaly—enlargement of the heart
12. hematuria—blood in urine
13. uremia—high levels of urea (waste material) in the blood
14. necrosis—abnormal condition of death of cells
15. cryotherapy—treatment by application of cold (freezing temperature)

E. **Name the part of the body described in the following terms and give the meaning of each term:**

1. cholecystectomy _____

2. myalgia _____

3. neuralgia _____

4. nephrosis _____

5. colitis _____

6. myocardial ischemia _____

7. bronchoscopy _____

8. hysterectomy _____

9. laparoscopy _____

10. mammoplasty _____

11. axillary _____

12. pneumonia _____

13. pulmonary _____

14. renal _____

◆ **ANSWER KEY**
1. gallbladder (removal of the gallbladder)
2. muscle (muscle pain)
3. nerve (nerve pain)
4. kidney (abnormal condition of a kidney)
5. colon (inflammation of the colon)
6. heart muscle (holding back blood to heart muscle)
7. bronchial tubes (visual examination of a bronchial tube)
8. uterus (removal of the uterus)
9. abdomen (visual examination of the abdomen)
10. breast (surgical repair of the breast)
11. armpit (pertaining to the armpit)
12. lung (abnormal condition of the lung)
13. lung (pertaining to the lung)
14. kidney (pertaining to the kidney)

F. **Match the following procedures with their meanings given below:**

radiotherapy	tracheostomy	myelogram
amniocentesis	chemotherapy	rhinoplasty
laparoscopy	craniotomy	hemodialysis
colostomy	electroencephalography	laparotomy

1. Treatment with drugs: _____

2. Surgical repair of the nose: _____

3. Separation of waste (urea) from the blood: _____

4. Opening of the windpipe to the outside of the body: _____

5. Surgical puncture to remove fluid from the sac around the fetus: _____

6. Incision of the skull: _____

7. Visual (endoscopic) examination of the abdomen: _____

8. Treatment with x-rays: _____

9. Record (x-ray) of the spinal cord: _____

10. Opening of the colon to the outside of the body: _____

11. Process of recording the electricity in the brain: _____

12. Incision of the abdomen (abdominal wall): _____

◆ **ANSWER KEY**

1. chemotherapy	7. laparoscopy
2. rhinoplasty	8. radiotherapy
3. hemodialysis	9. myelogram
4. tracheostomy	10. colostomy
5. amniocentesis	11. electroencephalography
6. craniotomy	12. laparotomy

G. Match the following abnormal conditions with their descriptions below:

atherosclerosis	cardiomyopathy	hepatomegaly
carcinoma	uremia	nephrosis
myocardial infarction	septicemia	adenoma
hematuria	sarcoma	cerebrovascular accident

1. Malignant tumor of connective tissue: _____

2. Benign tumor of a gland: _____

3. Heart attack (area of dead tissue in heart muscle): _____

4. Hardening of arteries by collection of plaque: _____

5. Stroke (blood vessels in the brain are damaged): _____

6. Disease condition of heart muscle (not a heart attack): _____

7. Abnormal condition of the kidney: _____

8. Blood infection: _____

9. Blood in the urine: _____

10. Excessive urea in the blood: _____

11. Cancerous tumor (of epithelial or surface tissues): _____

12. Enlargement of the liver: _____

◆ **ANSWER KEY**

1. sarcoma	7. nephrosis
2. adenoma	8. septicemia
3. myocardial infarction	9. hematuria
4. atherosclerosis	10. uremia
5. cerebrovascular accident	11. carcinoma
6. cardiomyopathy	12. hepatomegaly

H. What part of the body is inflamed?

1. neuritis _____

2. arthritis _____

3. salpingitis _____

4. otitis _____

5. hepatitis _____

6. nephritis _____

7. esophagitis _____

8. laryngitis _____

9. encephalitis _____

10. osteitis _____

11. meningitis _____

12. bronchitis _____

13. rhinitis _____

14. peritonitis _____

15. vasculitis _____

16. mastitis _____

17. tonsillitis _____

18. colitis _____

19. pharyngitis _____

20. tracheitis _____

21. phlebitis _____

◆ **ANSWER KEY**

1. nerve
2. joint
3. fallopian tubes
4. ear
5. liver
6. kidney
7. esophagus
8. larynx (voice box)
9. brain
10. bone
11. meninges (membranes surrounding the brain and spinal cord)

12. bronchial tubes
13. nose
14. peritoneum
15. blood vessels
16. breast
17. tonsils
18. colon (large intestine)
19. throat (pharynx)
20. trachea (windpipe)
21. veins

I. Provide the terms for the following procedures:

1. Excision of the gallbladder _____

2. Excision of the appendix _____

3. Excision of a breast _____

4. Excision of the uterus _____

5. Excision of an ovary _____

6. Excision of the voice box _____

7. Excision of a kidney _____

8. Excision of a gland _____

9. Excision of the large intestine _____

10. Excision of a fallopian tube _____

11. Excision of tonsils _____

12. Incision of the skull _____

13. Incision of the abdomen _____

14. Incision of the chest _____

15. Opening of the windpipe to the outside of the body _____

16. Opening of the colon to the outside of the body _____

17. Surgical puncture of the chest _____

18. Surgical puncture of the sac around the fetus _____

19. Incision of a vein _____

20. Visual examination of the voice box _____

◆ **ANSWER KEY**

1. cholecystectomy
2. appendectomy
3. mastectomy
4. hysterectomy
5. oophorectomy
6. laryngectomy
7. nephrectomy
8. adenectomy
9. colectomy
10. salpingectomy
11. tonsillectomy
12. craniotomy
13. laparotomy
14. thoracotomy
15. tracheostomy
16. colostomy
17. thoracentesis
18. amniocentesis
19. phlebotomy
20. laryngoscopy

J. Select from the following to complete the following definitions:

adenoma   myoma   encephalopathy
hepatoma   myosarcoma   arthropathy
radiotherapy   osteoma   cardiomyopathy
adenocarcinoma   hematoma   neuropathy

1. Collection (mass) of blood _____

2. Tumor of muscle (benign) _____

3. Treatment using x-rays _____

4. Tumor of a gland (benign) _____

5. Tumor of bone (benign) _____

6. Cancerous tumor of glandular tissue _____

7. Malignant tumor (flesh tissue) of muscle _____

8. Tumor of the liver _____

9. Disease of joints _____

10. Disease of heart muscle _____

11. Disease of nerves _____

12. Disease of the brain _____

ANSWER KEY   1. hematoma   7. myosarcoma
              2. myoma   8. hepatoma
              3. radiotherapy   9. arthropathy
              4. adenoma   10. cardiomyopathy
              5. osteoma   11. neuropathy
              6. adenocarcinoma   12. encephalopathy

K. Circle the term that best completes the meaning of the sentences in the following medical vignettes:

1. Nora felt a lump in her breast and immediately scheduled an x-ray exam called a(an) **(angiogram, bronchoscopy, mammogram).** The examination showed a stellate (star-shaped) mass that on biopsy revealed an infiltrating ductal carcinoma. Nora elected to have her breast removed and underwent **(hysterectomy, mastectomy, salpingectomy),** although her physician gave her the option of having lumpectomy followed by **(cryotherapy, thoracotomy, radiotherapy).**

2. In addition to her surgery, Nora had an **(axillary, inguinal, esophageal)** lymph node dissection to determine if the cancer had spread. Fortunately, this procedure revealed no evidence of metastatic disease in 10 sampled lymph nodes.

3. Sylvia had irregular bleeding in between her periods. She was 50 years old and beginning to undergo menopause. On pelvic exam, Dr. Hawk felt a large, lobulated uterus. A biopsy revealed fibroids, a condition known as **(multiple myeloma, hematoma, leiomyoma).** The doctor suggested a total abdominal **(gastrectomy, hysterectomy, cholecystectomy)** and bilateral salpingo- **(tonsillectomy, adenoidectomy, oophorectomy).**

4. Victoria had never been comfortable with the bump on her nose. She saw a plastic surgeon who performed a(an) **(mammoplasty, rhinoplasty, angioplasty).**

5. Sam was experiencing cramps, diarrhea, and a low-grade fever. He was diagnosed with ulcerative **(colitis, meningitis, laryngitis)** and had several bouts of **(uremia, menorrhagia, septicemia)** caused by inflammation and rupture of the bowel wall.

6. Bill was experiencing chest pain every time he climbed a flight of stairs. He went to his doctor who did a(an) **(myelogram, angiogram, dialysis)** and discovered **(adenocarcinoma, nephrosis, atherosclerosis)** in one of his coronary arteries. The doctor recommended a procedure called **(angioplasty, thoracentesis, amniocentesis).** This would prevent further **(otalgia, ischemia, neuralgia)** and help Bill avoid a **(peritoneal, vascular, myocardial)** infarction, or heart attack, in the future.

◆ **ANSWER KEY** 1. mammogram, mastectomy, radiotherapy
2. axillary
3. leiomyoma, hysterectomy, oophorectomy
4. rhinoplasty
5. colitis, septicemia
6. angiogram, atherosclerosis, angioplasty, ischemia, myocardial

V. REVIEW

Write the meanings for the following word parts, and don't forget to check your answers.

SUFFIXES

SUFFIX	MEANING	SUFFIX	MEANING
1. -al		15. -megaly	
2. -algia		16. -oma	
3. -ar		17. -osis	
4. -ary		18. -pathy	
5. -centesis		19. -plasty	
6. -eal		20. -rrhage	
7. -ectomy		21. -rrhagia	
8. -emia		22. -rrhea	
9. -gram		23. -sclerosis	
10. -graphy		24. -scopy	
11. -ia		25. -stomy	
12. -ic		26. -therapy	
13. -itis		27. -tomy	
14. -lysis		28. -uria	

COMBINING FORMS

COMBINING FORM	MEANING	COMBINING FORM	MEANING
1. aden/o		3. angi/o	
2. amni/o		4. arteri/o	

5. arthr/o _____

6. ather/o _____

7. axill/o _____

8. bronch/o _____

9. carcin/o _____

10. cardi/o _____

11. chem/o _____

12. cholecyst/o _____

13. chron/o _____

14. col/o _____

15. crani/o _____

16. cry/o _____

17. cyst/o _____

18. encephal/o _____

19. erythr/o _____

20. esophag/o _____

21. hemat/o _____

22. hepat/o _____

23. hyster/o _____

24. inguin/o _____

25. isch/o _____

26. lapar/o _____

27. laryng/o _____

28. leuk/o _____

29. mamm/o _____

30. mast/o _____

31. men/o _____

32. mening/o _____

33. my/o _____

34. myel/o _____

35. necr/o _____

36. nephr/o _____

37. neur/o _____

38. oophor/o _____

39. oste/o _____

40. ot/o _____

41. pelv/o _____

42. peritone/o _____

43. phleb/o _____

44. pneumon/o _____

45. pulmon/o _____

46. radi/o _____

47. ren/o _____

48. rhin/o _____

49. salping/o _____

50. sarc/o _____

51. septic/o   _____

52. thorac/o   _____

53. tonsill/o   _____

54. trache/o   _____

55. ur/o   _____

56. vascul/o   _____

SUFFIXES

◆ **ANSWER KEY**

1. pertaining to
2. pain
3. pertaining to
4. pertaining to
5. surgical puncture to remove fluid
6. pertaining to
7. removal, resection, excision
8. blood condition
9. record
10. process of recording
11. condition
12. pertaining to
13. inflammation
14. separation, breakdown, destruction
15. enlargement
16. tumor, mass
17. abnormal condition
18. disease condition
19. surgical repair
20. bursting forth of blood
21. bursting forth of blood
22. flow, discharge
23. hardening
24. visual examination
25. opening
26. treatment
27. incision
28. urine condition

COMBINING FORMS

◆ **ANSWER KEY**

1. gland
2. amnion
3. blood vessel
4. artery
5. joint
6. plaque, collection of fatty material
7. armpit
8. bronchial tubes
9. cancerous
10. heart
11. drug, chemical
12. gallbladder
13. time
14. colon (large intestine)
15. skull
16. cold
17. urinary bladder
18. brain
19. red
20. esophagus
21. blood
22. liver
23. uterus
24. groin
25. to hold back
26. abdomen
27. larynx (voice box)
28. white
29. breast
30. breast
31. menstruation

32. meninges	45. lungs
33. muscle	46. x-rays
34. spinal cord or bone marrow	47. kidney
35. death	48. nose
36. kidney	49. fallopian tube
37. nerve	50. flesh
38. ovary	51. pertaining to infection
39. bone	52. chest
40. ear	53. tonsils
41. hip bone	54. trachea (windpipe)
42. peritoneum	55. urine, urinary tract
43. vein	56. blood vessel
44. lungs	

VI. PRONUNCIATION OF TERMS

The terms that you have learned in this chapter are presented here with their pronunciations. The capitalized letters in boldface are the accented syllable. Pronounce each word out loud, then write the meaning in the space provided.

TERM	PRONUNCIATION	MEANING
acute	ah-**KUT**	
adenocarcinoma	ah-deh-no-kar-sih-**NO**-mah	
adenoma	ah-deh-**NO**-mah	
amniocentesis	am-ne-o-sen-**TE**-sis	
angiography	an-je-**OG**-rah-fe	
angioplasty	**AN**-je-o-plas-te	
arteriosclerosis	ar-ter-e-o-skle-**RO**-sis	
arthralgia	ar-**THRAL**-je-ah	
arthropathy	ar-**THROP**-ah-the	
atherosclerosis	ah-theh-ro-skle-**RO**-sis	

axillary	**AKS**-ih-lar-e _____
bronchitis	brong-**KI**-tis _____
bronchoscopy	brong-**KOS**-ko-pe _____
carcinoma	kar-sih-**NO**-mah _____
cardiomegaly	kar-de-o-**MEG**-ah-le _____
cardiomyopathy	kar-de-o-mi-**OP**-ah-the _____
chemotherapy	ke-mo-**THER**-ah-pe _____
cholecystectomy	ko-le-sis-**TEK**-to-me _____
chronic	**KRON**-ik _____
colitis	ko-**LI**-tis _____
colostomy	ko-**LOS**-to-me _____
craniotomy	kra-ne-**OT**-o-me _____
cystitis	sis-**TI**-tis _____
dialysis	di-**AL**-ih-sis _____
electroencephalography	e-lek-tro-en-sef-ah-**LOG**-rah-fe _____
encephalopathy	en-sef-ah-**LOP**-ah-the _____
erythrocytosis	eh-rith-ro-si-**TO**-sis _____
esophageal	e-sof-ah-**JE**-al _____
esophagitis	e-sof-ah-**JI**-tis _____
hematoma	he-mah-**TO**-mah _____
hematuria	he-mah-**TUR**-e-ah _____
hemorrhage	**HEM**-or-ij _____

hysterectomy	his-teh-**REK**-to-me _____
infarction	in-**FARK**-shun _____
inguinal	**ING**-gwi-nal _____
ischemia	is-**KE**-me-ah _____
laparoscopy	lap-ah-**ROS**-ko-pe _____
laparotomy	lap-ah-**ROT**-o-me _____
laryngitis	lah-rin-**JI**-tis _____
laryngoscopy	lah-rin-**GOS**-ko-pe _____
leukemia	lu-**KE**-me-ah _____
leukocytosis	lu-ko-si-**TO**-sis _____
mammogram	**MAM**-o-gram _____
mammography	mam-**MOG**-rah-fe _____
mammoplasty	**MAM**-o-plas-te _____
mastectomy	mas-**TEK**-to-me _____
meningitis	men-in-**JI**-tis _____
menorrhagia	men-or-**RA**-jah _____
menorrhea	men-o-**RE**-ah _____
myalgia	mi-**AL**-jah _____
myelogram	**MI**-eh-lo-gram _____
myeloma	mi-eh-**LO**-mah _____
myocardial	mi-o-**KAR**-de-al _____
myoma	mi-**O**-mah _____

myosarcoma	mi-o-sar-**KO**-mah _____
necrosis	neh-**KRO**-sis _____
nephrosis	neh-**FRO**-sis _____
neuralgia	nu-**RAL**-jah _____
oophorectomy	o-of-o-**REK**-to-me or oo-for-**REK**-to-me _____
otalgia	o-**TAL**-jah _____
pelvic	**PEL**-vik _____
peritoneal	per-ih-to-**NE**-al _____
phlebitis	fleh-**BI**-tis _____
phlebotomy	fleh-**BOT**-o-me _____
pneumonia	noo-**MO**-ne-ah _____
pulmonary	**PUL**-mo-ner-re _____
radiotherapy	ra-de-o-**THER**-ah-pe _____
renal	**RE**-nal _____
rhinoplasty	**RI**-no-plas-te _____
rhinorrhea	ri-no-**RE**-ah _____
salpingectomy	sal-ping-**JEK**-to-me _____
septicemia	sep-tih-**SE**-me-ah _____
thoracentesis	tho-rah-sen-**TE**-sis _____
tonsillectomy	ton-sih-**LEK**-to-me _____
tracheostomy	tra-ke-**OS**-to-me _____
uremia	u-**RE**-me-ah _____
vascular	**VAS**-ku-lar _____

VII. PRACTICAL APPLICATIONS

A. Match the procedure in Column I with an abnormal condition it treats or diagnoses in Column II:

| COLUMN I | | COLUMN II |
| PROCEDURE | | DIAGNOSIS |

1. angioplasty   _____

2. mammoplasty   _____

3. cholecystectomy   _____

4. tonsillectomy   _____

5. dialysis   _____

6. hysterectomy   _____

7. thoracentesis   _____

8. oophorectomy   _____

9. tracheostomy   _____

10. arthroscopy   _____

A. Uterine adenocarcinoma

B. Ligament tear of the patella (knee cap)

C. Ovarian cyst

D. Blockage of the windpipe

E. Renal failure

F. Absence of a breast (post-mastectomy)

G. Pleural effusion (collection of fluid)

H. Coronary atherosclerosis

I. Gallbladder calculi (stones)

J. Pharyngeal lymph node enlargement

ANSWER KEY

| 1. H | 2. F | 3. I | 4. J | 5. E |
| 6. A | 7. G | 8. C | 9. D | 10. B |

B. Match the symptom or abnormal condition in Column I with the organ or tissue affected in Column II:

COLUMN I *SYMPTOM OR ABNORMAL CONDITION*	COLUMN II *ORGAN OR TISSUE*
1. colitis _____	a. Uterus
2. phlebitis _____	b. Ear
3. menorrhagia _____	c. Bone marrow
4. myocardial ischemia _____	d. Coronary arteries
5. otalgia _____	e. Large bowel
6. uremia _____	f. Spinal cord or brain
7. meningitis _____	g. Vein
8. leukemia _____	h. Kidney

◆ **ANSWER KEY** 1. e   2. g   3. a   4. d
                  5. b   6. h   7. f   8. c

PREFIXES

CHAPTER SECTIONS

CHAPTER OBJECTIVES

- To identify and define common prefixes used in medical terms
- To analyze, spell, and pronounce medical terms that contain prefixes

I. INTRODUCTION

This chapter reviews the prefixes that were introduced in Chapter 1 and covers new prefixes as well. The list of Combining Forms and Suffixes in Section II will help you understand the Prefixes and Terminology in Section III. Complete the Exercises in Section IV and the Review in Section V. Don't forget to check your answers! The answers to the exercises are placed directly after the questions so that you can use them easily. The Pronunciation of Terms in Section VI is your final review of the terminology in this chapter.

II. COMBINING FORMS AND SUFFIXES

COMBINING FORM	MEANING
abdomin/o	abdomen
an/o	anus (opening of the digestive tract to the outside of the body)
bi/o	life
cardi/o	heart
carp/o	carpals (wrist bones)
cis/o	to cut
cost/o	ribs
crani/o	skull
cutane/o	skin
dur/o	dura mater (outermost meningeal membrane surrounding the brain and spinal cord)
gen/o	to produce, to begin
glyc/o	sugar
hemat/o	blood
later/o	side
men/o	menses (monthly discharge of blood from the lining of the uterus)
nat/i	birth
neur/o	nerve
norm/o	rule, order
oste/o	bone
peritone/o	peritoneum (membrane surrounding the organs in the abdomen)
plas/o	formation, growth, development
ren/o	kidney
scapul/o	scapula (shoulder blade)
son/o	sound
thyroid/o	thyroid gland
top/o	to put, place, position

troph/o	development, nourishment
urethr/o	urethra (tube leading from the bladder to the outside of the body)
uter/o	uterus
ven/o	vein
vertebr/o	vertebra (backbone)

SUFFIX	MEANING
-al	pertaining to
-ation	process, condition
-cision	process of cutting
-crine	secretion
-dipsia	thirst
-emia	blood condition
-gen	to produce
-graphy	process of recording
-ia	condition, process
-ic	pertaining to
-ine	pertaining to
-ism	condition, process
-lapse	to fall, slide
-lysis	loosening, breakdown, separation, destruction
-mission	to send
-mortem	death
-oma	tumor, mass
-ous	pertaining to
-partum	birth
-pathy	disease condition
-phagia	to eat, swallow
-phasia	to speak
-plasm	formation
-plegia	paralysis
-pnea	breathing
-rrhea	flow, discharge
-scopy	process of visual examination
-section	to cut
-stasis	to stand, place, stop, control
-tension	pressure
-thesis	to put, place
-tic	pertaining to
-um	structure
-uria	urine condition
-y	process, condition

III. PREFIXES AND TERMINOLOGY

PREFIX	MEANING	TERMINOLOGY	MEANING

a-, an-   no, not, without   apnea _____

aphasia _____
A stroke on the left side of the brain can produce this condition.

atrophy _____
Disuse of a muscle can result in muscular atrophy. Muscles shrink as cells decrease in size.

anemia _____
Anemia is a condition in which there is a lower-than-normal number of red blood cells or a decrease in hemoglobin in the cells. Table 4-1 lists some of the different forms of anemia.

amenorrhea _____

ab-   away from   abnormal _____

ad-   toward, near   adrenal glands _____
Adrenal glands are also called _suprarenal_ (SUPRA- means "above") glands. See Figure 4-1.

ana-   up, apart   analysis _____
A _urinalysis_ (urine + analysis) is a separation of urine to determine its contents.

ante-   before, forward   ante partum _____

ante mortem _____

anti-   against   antibody _____
An antibody is a protein made by white blood cells; literally, a "body" working "against" foreign substances.

TABLE 4-1 ◆ Anemias	
aplastic anemia	Bone marrow fails to produce red blood cells (erythrocytes), white blood cells (leukocytes), and clotting cells (platelets).
hemolytic anemia	Red blood cells are destroyed (-LYTIC), and bone marrow cannot compensate for their loss. This condition can be hereditary or acquired (after infection or chemoherapy) or can occur when the immune system acts against normal red blood cells (autoimmune condition).
iron deficiency anemia	Low or absent iron levels lead to low hemoglobin concentration or deficiency of red blood cells.
pernicious anemia	The mucous membrane of the stomach fails to produce a factor (intrinsic factor) that is necessary for the absorption of vitamin B_{12} and the proper formation of red blood cells.
sickle cell anemia	Erythrocytes assume an abnormal crescent or sickle shape; it is caused by the inheritance of an abnormal type of hemoglobin. The sickle-shaped cells clump together, causing clots that block blood vessels.

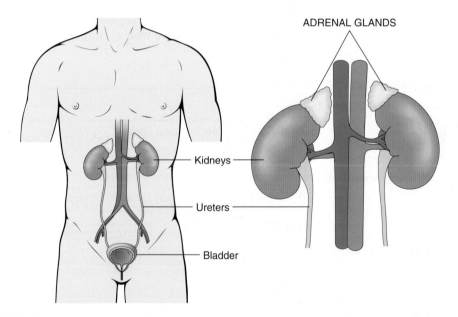

FIGURE 4-1

Adrenal glands. These two endocrine glands are above each kidney. (From Chabner D-E: *The Language of Medicine,* ed 6, Philadelphia, 2001, WB Saunders.)

antigen _____

Antigens are foreign substances, such as bacteria and viruses. When antigens enter the body, they stimulate white blood cells to produce antibodies that act against the antigens. Think of the ANTI- in *antigen* as standing for antibody, so that *antigen* means "to produce (-GEN) antibodies."

antibiotic _____

Antibiotics differ from antibodies in that they are produced *outside* the body by primitive plants called molds. Examples of antibiotics are penicillin and erythromycin.

bi-	two, both	bilateral _____
brady-	slow	bradycardia _____
con-	with, together	congenital _____

A congenital anomaly is an irregularity (anomaly) present at birth. Examples are webbed fingers and toes and heart defects.

dia-	through, complete	diarrhea _____

dialysis _____
-LYSIS means "separation" here.

dys-	bad, painful, difficult, abnormal	dyspnea _____

dysphagia _____

dysplasia _____

dysmenorrhea _____

dysuria _____

ec-	out, outside	ectopic pregnancy _____

Figure 4-2 shows possible sites of ectopic pregnancies. Figure 4-3 indicates uterine levels in a normal pregnancy.

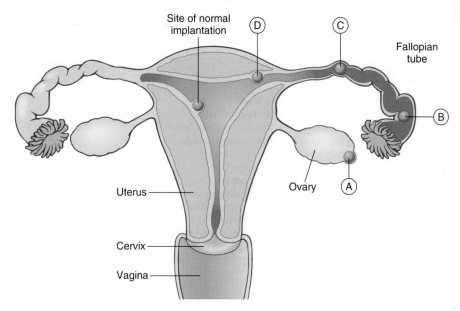

FIGURE 4-2

Ectopic pregnancy. A, B, C, and **D** are ectopic sites. The fallopian tube is the most common site for ectopic pregnancies (95%), but they can also occur on the ovary or on the surface of the peritoneum. Normal implantation takes place on the inner lining (endometrium) of the uterus.

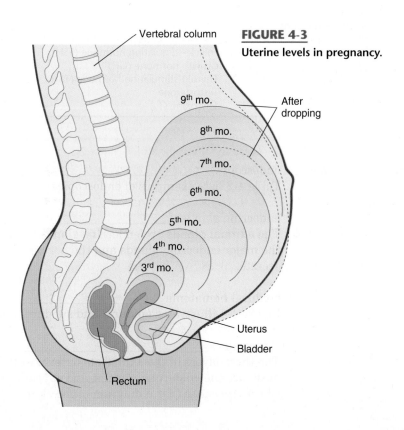

FIGURE 4-3

Uterine levels in pregnancy.

TABLE 4-2 ◆ Endoscopies	
arthroscopy	Visual examination of a joint
bronchoscopy	Visual examination of the bronchial tubes
colonoscopy	Visual examination of the colon (large intestine)
cystoscopy	Visual examination of the urinary bladder
esophagoscopy	Visual examination of the esophagus
gastroscopy	Visual examination of the stomach
hysteroscopy	Visual examination of the uterus
laparoscopy	Visual examination of the abdomen
laryngoscopy	Visual examination of the larynx (voice box)
mediastinoscopy	Visual examination of the mediastinum
proctosigmoidoscopy	Visual examination of the rectum and sigmoid colon
sigmoidoscopy	Visual examination of the sigmoid colon (lower, S-shaped part of the large intestine)

TABLE 4-3 ◆ Major Endocrine Glands and Selected Hormones	
GLAND	HORMONES
adrenal glands	Adrenalin (epinephrine)
ovaries	Estrogen
	Progesterone
pancreas	Insulin
parathyroid glands	Parathyroid hormone (PTH)
pituitary gland	Adrenocorticotrophic hormone (ACTH)
	Follicle-stimulating hormone (FSH)
	Growth hormone (GH)
	Thyroid-stimulating hormone (TSH)
testes	Testosterone
thyroid gland	Thyroxine (T_4)

endo-	within, in, inner	endoscopy _____ Table 4-2 lists examples of endoscopies. endocrine glands _____ The adrenal glands are endocrine glands. Table 4-3 lists the major endocrine glands and the hormones they secrete.
epi-	above, upon	epidural hematoma _____ Figure 4-4 illustrates epidural and subdural hematomas. epidermis _____ The three layers of the skin, from outermost to innermost, are the epidermis, dermis, and subcutaneous layer. Check *Appendix I* for a diagram of the skin.

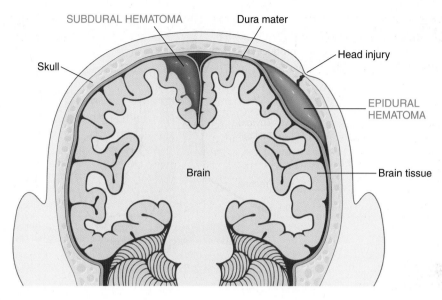

FIGURE 4-4

Epidural and subdural hematomas. The dura mater is the outermost of the three meninges (membranes) around the brain and spinal cord.

ex-	out	excision _____
extra-	outside of	extrahepatic _____
hemi-	half	hemigastrectomy _____

hemiplegia _____
One side of the body is paralyzed; usually caused by a cerebral vascular accident or a brain lesion, such as a tumor. The paralysis occurs on the side opposite the brain disorder.

| hyper- | excessive, above | hyperthyroidism _____ |

Figure 4-5 shows the position of the thyroid gland in the neck.

hypertrophy _____
Cells increase in size, not in number. The opposite of hypertrophy is *atrophy* (cells shrink in size).

FIGURE 4-5

Thyroid gland, located in the front of the trachea in the neck. The thyroid gland produces too much hormone in hyperthyroidism.

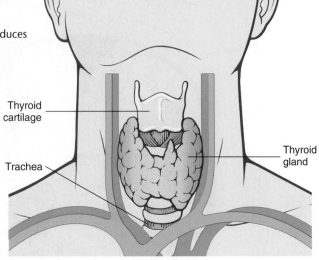

Thyroid cartilage

Trachea

Thyroid gland

hypertension _____

Risk factors that contribute to high blood pressure are increasing age, smoking, obesity, heredity, and a stressful life style.

hyperglycemia _____

Also known as diabetes mellitus. *Mellitus* means "sweet." Insulin is either not secreted or improperly utilized so that sugar accumulates in the bloodstream and "spills over" into the urine.

hypo-   below, deficient   hypoglycemia _____

Overproduction of insulin or an overdose (from outside the body—exogenously) of insulin can lead to hypoglycemia, as glucose is removed from the blood at an increased rate.

in-   in, into   incision _____

inter-   between   intervertebral _____

intra-   within   intrauterine _____

intravenous _____

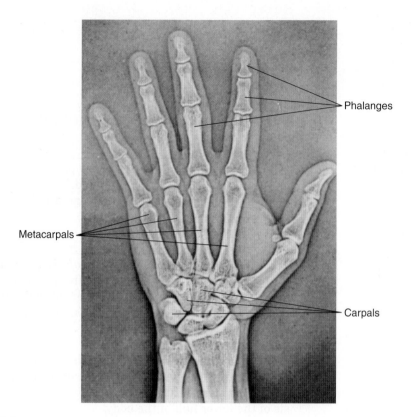

FIGURE 4-6

Metacarpals. This x-ray film of a hand shows metacarpals, carpals (wrist bones), and phalanges (finger bones).

mal-	bad	malignant _____ -IGNANT comes from the Latin *ignis,* meaning a "fire." A malignant tumor is a cancerous growth. A *benign* tumor (*ben* means "good") is a non-cancerous growth.
meta-	change, beyond	metastasis _____ This term literally means a "change of place" (-STASIS). It is the spread of a cancerous tumor from its original place to a secondary location in the body. metacarpals _____ The carpal bones are the wrist bones, and the metacarpals are the hand bones, which are "beyond the wrist." See the x-ray picture of the hand in Figure 4-6.

neo-	new	neoplasm _____
		neoplastic _____
		neonatal _____

Neonates who are born prematurely are often treated in the neonatal intensive care unit (NICU). See Figure 4-7.

para-	beside, near, along the side of	parathyroid glands _____

Figure 4-8 shows the position of the parathyroid glands on the back side of the thyroid gland. The parathyroid glands are endocrine glands that regulate the amount of calcium in bones and in the blood.

paralysis _____

This term came from the Greek *paralyikos,* meaning "one whose side was loose or weak," as after a stroke. Now it means a loss of movement in any part of the body caused by a break in the connection between nerve and muscle.

paraplegia _____

-PLEGIA means "paralysis," and this term originally meant "paralysis of any limb or side of the body." Since the nineteenth century, however, it has indicated paralysis of the lower half of the body.

peri-	surrounding	periosteum _____
		perianal _____
poly-	many, much	polyuria _____
		polyneuropathy _____
		polydipsia _____

Symptoms of diabetes mellitus are polyuria and polydipsia.

post-	after, behind	post partum _____
		post mortem _____
pre-	before	precancerous _____

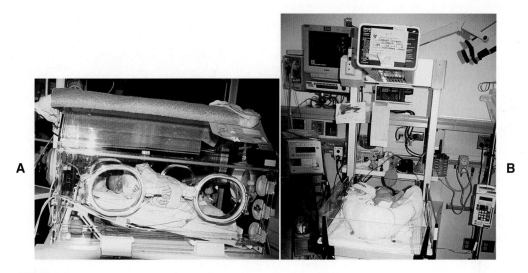

FIGURE 4-7

Neonates in the neonatal intensive care unit (NICU). A, Benjamin Oliver Chabner, born May 22, 2001, at 32 weeks (8 weeks premature). **B,** Samuel August Thompson, born August 13, 2001, at 36 weeks. "Gust" needed an endotracheal tube through which he received surfactant, a substance necessary to inflate his lungs. Both babies are now healthy and are a delight to their grandmother.

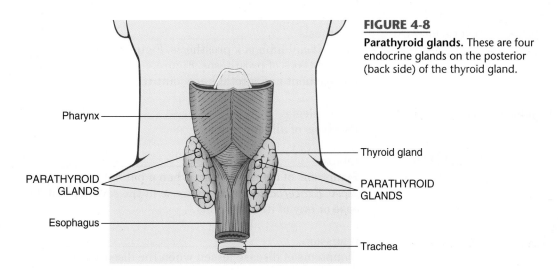

FIGURE 4-8

Parathyroid glands. These are four endocrine glands on the posterior (back side) of the thyroid gland.

Pharynx

PARATHYROID
GLANDS

Esophagus

Thyroid gland

PARATHYROID
GLANDS

Trachea

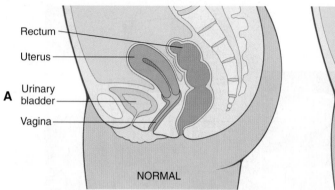
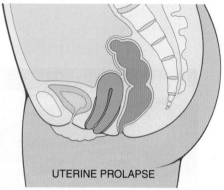

Rectum
Uterus
A
Urinary bladder
Vagina

NORMAL   UTERINE PROLAPSE

B

FIGURE 4-9

Prolapsed uterus is shown in **B**. Normally, the uterus is tilted forward above the bladder (**A**).

		prenatal _____
pro-	before, forward	prolapse _____ -LAPSE means "to slide." Figure 4-9 shows both the normal position of the uterus and its position when prolapsed.
pros-	before, forward	prosthesis _____ An artificial limb is a prosthesis. Figure 4-10 illustrates several types of prostheses. Figure 4-11 shows a total hip replacement and a total knee joint replacement.
quadri-	four	quadriplegia _____ Paralysis of all four limbs.
re-	back, behind	relapse _____ Symptoms of disease return when a patient has a relapse. *Exacerbation* is an increase in the severity of a disease or any of its symptoms. remission _____ Symptoms of disease lessen when the disease goes into remission. resection _____

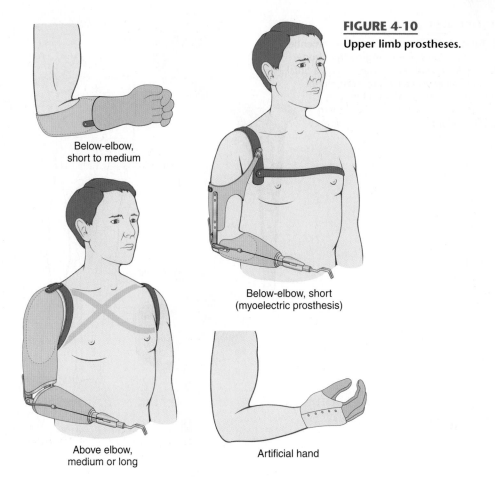

FIGURE 4-10
Upper limb prostheses.

Below-elbow,
short to medium

Below-elbow, short
(myoelectric prosthesis)

Above elbow,
medium or long

Artificial hand

retro-	back, behind	retroperitoneal _____
		The kidneys and adrenal glands are retroperitoneal organs.
sub-	under, less than	subcostal _____
		subcutaneous _____
		subtotal _____
		A subtotal gastrectomy is a partial resection of the stomach.

FIGURE 4-11

A, Total hip joint replacement. A cementless prosthesis allows porous ingrowth of bone. **B,** Total knee joint replacement using a tibial metal retainer and a femoral component. The femoral component is chosen individually for each person according to the amount of healthy bone present.

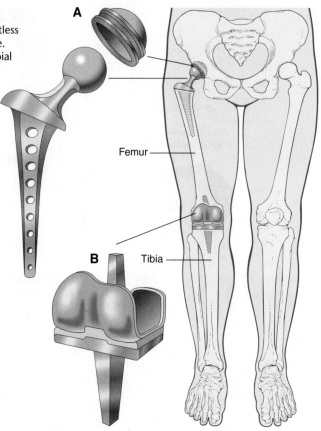

Femur

Tibia

subscapular _____
The scapula is the shoulder bone. Figure 4-12 shows its location.

syn-   with, together   syndrome _____
-DROME means "to run" or "occur." Syndromes are groups of symptoms or signs of illness that occur together. Table 4-4 gives examples of syndromes.

tachy-   fast   tachycardia _____

tachypnea _____

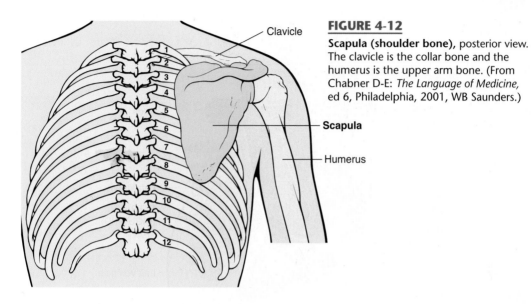

FIGURE 4-12

Scapula (shoulder bone), posterior view. The clavicle is the collar bone and the humerus is the upper arm bone. (From Chabner D-E: *The Language of Medicine,* ed 6, Philadelphia, 2001, WB Saunders.)

Labels: Clavicle, **Scapula**, Humerus

TABLE 4-4	Syndromes

acquired immunodeficiency syndrome (AIDS)	Symptoms are severe infections, malignancy (Kaposi sarcoma and lymphoma), fever, malaise (discomfort), and gastrointestinal disturbances. It is caused by a virus that damages lymphocytes (white blood cells).
Barlow syndrome (mitral valve prolapse)	Symptoms are abnormal sounds (murmurs) heard from the chest when listening with a stethoscope. These murmurs indicate that the mitral valve is not closing properly. Chest pain, dyspnea (difficult breathing), and fatigue are other symptoms.
carpal tunnel syndrome	Symptoms are pain, tingling, burning, and numbness of the hand. A nerve leading to the hand is compressed by connective tissue fibers in the wrist.
Down syndrome	Symptoms include mental retardation, flat face with a short nose, slanted eyes, broad hands and feet, stubby fingers, and protruding lower lip. The syndrome occurs when an extra chromosome is present in each cell of the body.
toxic shock syndrome	Symptoms are high fever, vomiting, diarrhea, rash, hypotension (low blood pressure), and shock. It is caused by a bacterial infection in the vagina of menstruating women using superabsorbent tampons.

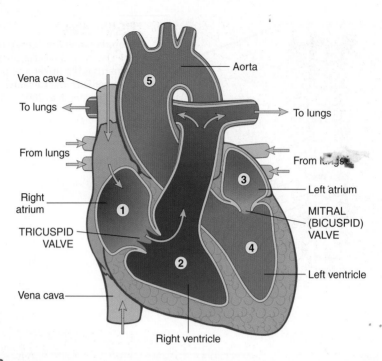

FIGURE 4-13

Tricuspid and mitral valves of the heart. Blood enters the *right atrium* of the heart *(1)* from the big veins (venae cavae) and passes through the *tricuspid valve* to the *right ventricle (2)*. Blood then travels to the *lungs* where it loses carbon dioxide (a gaseous waste) and picks up oxygen. Blood returns to the heart into the *left atrium (3)* and passes through the mitral (bicuspid) valve to the *left ventricle (4)*. It is then pumped from the left ventricle out of the heart into the largest artery, the *aorta (5)*, which carries the blood to all parts of the body.

trans-	across, through	transabdominal _____
		transurethral _____
tri-	three	tricuspid valve _____

-CUSPID means "pointed end," as of a spear. The tricuspid valve is on the right side of the heart. The mitral or bicuspid valve is on the left side of the heart. Figure 4-13 shows the location of both valves and indicates the pathway of blood through the heart.

ultra-	beyond	ultrasonography _____

Figure 4-14 shows an ultrasonogram (sonogram) of a fetus.

uni-	one	unilateral _____

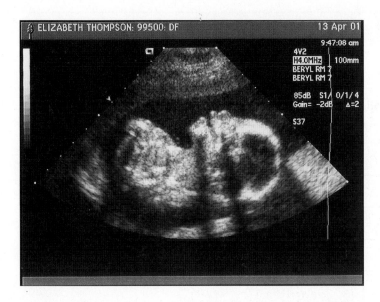

FIGURE 4-14

Ultrasonogram of my grandson, Samuel August Thompson as a 19-week-old fetus. (Courtesy Dr. Elizabeth Chabner Thompson.)

IV. EXERCISES AND ANSWERS

A. Match the prefix in Column I with its meaning in Column II:

COLUMN I		COLUMN II
1. dia-	____	A. across, through
2. neo-	____	B. no, not, without
3. peri-	____	C. bad, painful, difficult
4. an-	____	D. new
5. brady-	____	E. near, along the side of
6. uni-	____	F. surrounding
7. trans-	____	G. through, complete
8. ultra-	____	H. one
9. para-	____	I. slow
10. dys-	____	J. beyond

B. Give meanings for the following prefixes:

1. meta- _____

2. ana- _____

3. a-, an- _____

4. bi- _____

5. inter- _____

6. para- _____

7. in- _____

8. mal- _____

9. anti- _____

10. con- _____

C. Select from the prefixes given in Column II to match meanings in Column I. Write the prefix in the space provided next to its meaning.

COLUMN I		COLUMN II
1. bad, painful, difficult	_____	hyper-
2. out, outside	_____	meta-
		pro-, pros-

3. away from   _____   intra-

4. fast   _____   syn-

     ab-

5. before, forward   _____   re-, retro-

6. back, behind   _____   hypo-

     uni-

7. less than, below   _____   dia-

8. three   _____   tachy-

9. together, with   _____   ec-

     dys-

10. within   _____   ad-

     inter-

     tri-

◆ **ANSWER KEY**

1. dys-	6. re-, retro-
2. ec-	7. hypo-
3. ab-	8. tri-
4. tachy-	9. syn-
5. pro-, pros-	10. intra-

D. Give the meaning of each of the following prefixes:

1. ante- _____

2. ad- _____

3. brady- _____

4. endo- _____

5. epi- _____

6. post- _____

7. pre- _____

8. sub- _____

9. extra- _____

10. dia- _____

11. hemi- _____

12. quadri- _____

◆ ANSWER KEY	1. before, forward	7. before
	2. toward	8. beneath, less than
	3. slow	9. out, outside of
	4. within, in, inner	10. through, complete
	5. above, upon	11. half
	6. after, behind	12. four

E. Circle the correct meaning in each of the following:

1. Dys- and mal- both mean (outside, good, bad).

2. Hypo- and sub- both mean (under, above, outside).

3. Epi- and hyper- both mean (inside, beneath, above).

4. Con- and syn- both mean (apart, near, with).

5. Ultra- and meta- both mean (new, beyond, without).

6. Ante-, pre-, and pro- all mean (before, surrounding, between).

7. Ec- and extra- both mean (within, many, outside).

8. Endo-, intra-, and in- all mean (painful, within, through).

9. Post-, re-, and retro- all mean (behind, slow, together).

10. Uni- means (one, two, three).

11. Tri- means (one, two, three).

12. Bi- means (one, two, three).

◆ **ANSWER KEY**
1. bad	7. outside
2. under	8. within
3. above	9. behind
4. with	10. one
5. beyond	11. three
6. before	12. two

F. Complete each of the sentences below by selecting from the following list. The italicized words in each sentence should help you choose the correct term.

analysis	prenatal	atrophy	unilateral
dysmenorrhea	bradycardia	adrenal glands	extracranial
antibody	dyspnea	parathyroid glands	epidural hematoma
bilateral	metacarpal	hypertrophy	antigen

1. Two glands located *near* (toward) the kidneys are the _____.

2. People suffering from asthma often have *difficulty* breathing, which is known as

   _____.

3. A problem that only affects *one* side of the body is a(an) _____ defect.

4. Some people have a *slow* heart rhythm called _____.

5. A condition of *painful* menstrual discharge is called _____.

6. The bones that are *beyond* the wrist are the hand bones, or _____ bones.

7. A protein substance that is made by white blood cells to act *against* foreign

   microorganisms is called a(an) _____.

8. An injury to the *outside* of the skull would be known as a(an) _____ lesion.

9. Four glands located in the neck region *near* (posterior to) another endocrine gland

   are _____.

10. Taking a substance *apart* to understand what it contains is called a(an)

    _____.

11. A collection of blood located *above* the outermost layer of membranes surrounding

the brain is called a(an) _____.

12. A problem that occurs *before* the birth of an infant is called _____.

13. *Excessive* development (individual cells increase in size) of an organ is known

as _____.

14. When a part of the body is not used, *no* development occurs, and the body shrinks in

size, which is known as _____.

15. A problem affecting *both* sides of the body is called a(an) _____ defect.

◆ **ANSWER KEY**

1. adrenal glands
2. dyspnea
3. unilateral
4. bradycardia
5. dysmenorrhea
6. metacarpal
7. antibody
8. extracranial
9. parathyroid glands
10. analysis
11. epidural hematoma
12. prenatal
13. hypertrophy
14. atrophy
15. bilateral

G. Underline the prefix in each term, and give the meaning of the entire term:

1. dysuria _____

2. hypoglycemia _____

3. polydipsia _____

4. syndrome _____

5. precancerous _____

6. apnea _____

7. anemia _____

8. endoscopy _____

9. prosthesis _____

10. antibiotic _____

11. hemiplegia _____

12. dysphagia _____

13. polyneuropathy _____

14. intravenous _____

◆ **ANSWER KEY**
1. dysuria—painful urination
2. hypoglycemia—low levels of sugar in the blood
3. polydipsia—condition of excess thirst
4. syndrome—group of symptoms that occur together, characterizing an abnormal condition
5. precancerous—before cancer
6. apnea—not breathing
7. anemia—literally, no blood; actually a decrease in red blood cells or in the hemoglobin within the cells
8. endoscopy—process of viewing within the body (an endoscope is used)
9. prosthesis—to put or place before (an artificial body part)
10. antibiotic—pertaining to a substance that acts against bacterial or germ life
11. hemiplegia—paralysis of one half of the body
12. dysphagia—difficult swallowing
13. polyneuropathy—disease of many nerves
14. intravenous—pertaining to within a vein

H. Define the following terms that describe an organ, tissue, or space in the body:

1. subscapular _____

2. intrauterine _____

3. periosteum _____

4. intervertebral _____

5. subcostal _____

6. transabdominal _____

7. perianal _____

8. extracranial _____

9. subcutaneous _____

10. retroperitoneal _____

◆ **ANSWER KEY**

1. pertaining to under the shoulder
2. pertaining to within the uterus
3. pertaining to surrounding the bone (this is a membrane surrounding the bone)
4. pertaining to between two vertebrae (a disc is an intervertebral structure)
5. pertaining to under a rib
6. pertaining to across the abdomen
7. pertaining to surrounding the anus
8. pertaining to outside the skull
9. pertaining to under the skin
10. pertaining to behind the peritoneum

I. **Choose a term from the following list to complete each of the sentences below:**

congenital	ectopic	subtotal	metastasis
transurethral	prosthesis	malignant	hyperthyroidism
tachycardia	ultrasonography	tricuspid	endocrine
dialysis	diarrhea	dysplasia	antigen

1. Enlargement of an endocrine gland in the neck can lead to _____.

2. An artificial limb is a(an) _____.

3. If the colon does not reabsorb the proper amount of water back into the bloodstream, _____ occurs.

4. An abnormally rapid heart beat is a _____.

5. Infection or abnormal ("bad") growth of cells on the uterine cervix can cause a condition known as cervical _____.

6. A test that shows the structure of organs in the abdomen by using sound waves is _____.

7. The spread of a cancerous tumor to a secondary place in the body is a(an) _____.

8. The process of filtering the waste materials from the blood using a machine that does the work of the kidneys is called _____.

9. The _____ valve is composed of three parts and is located on the right side of the heart between the upper and lower chambers.

10. A procedure to remove the prostate gland by cutting across (through) the urethra is a _____ resection of the prostate.

11. Cancerous growths are _____ neoplasms.

12. An abnormal condition that occurs at birth is a(an) _____ anomaly.

13. A gland that secretes hormones into the bloodstream is a(an) _____ gland.

14. A foreign organism, such as a virus or bacterium, that enters the body and stimulates white blood cells to make antibodies is a(an) _____.

15. An embryo that grows outside the uterus (extrauterine) is a(an) _____ pregnancy.

16. The doctors did not remove the whole organ; they did a partial or _____ resection.

J. Use the following terms to complete the sentences below:

transurethral	relapse	incision	analysis
prolapse	neoplastic	post partum	paralysis
neonatal	tachycardia	post mortem	anemia
remission	aphasia	ante partum	resection

1. Complete removal of Ms. Smith's stomach was necessary because of the presence of an adenocarcinoma. Dr. Nife performed the gastric _____.

2. After she had nine children, Ms. White's uterine walls became weak, causing her uterus to fall and _____ through her vagina.

3. The autopsy or _____ examination of a dead body is an important step in determining the cause of death.

4. After Mr. Puffer's heart attack, doctors were concerned because he continued to have a persistent, rapid, abnormal heart rhythm. They prescribed drugs called antiarrhythmics to treat his _____.

5. The special ward in the hospital devoted to newborn babies is known as the _____ unit.

6. Ms. Rose was pleased that she hadn't had symptoms of her malignant disease for the past six years. Her illness was in _____.

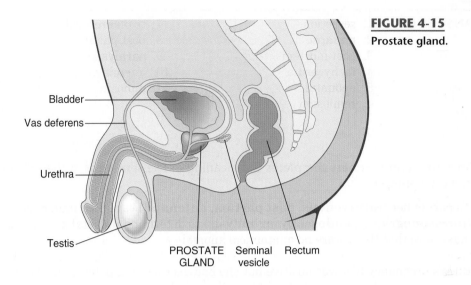

FIGURE 4-15
Prostate gland.

Bladder

Vas deferens

Urethra

Testis

PROSTATE GLAND

Seminal vesicle

Rectum

7. The operation to remove part of Mr. Jones' enlarged (hypertrophied) prostate gland involved placing a catheter through his urethra and removing pieces of the prostate through the tube. The surgery is called a _____ resection of the prostate gland (TURP). The prostate gland is located at the base of the bladder in males. See Figure 4-15.

8. Mr. M. Pathy was in a sad mood for several weeks after his wife had their first baby. He was experiencing a(an) _____ depression.

9. Ms. Smith's recent stroke left her with loss of muscle movement on the right side of her body, also called right-sided _____.

10. Excessive bleeding or lack of iron in the diet can lead to a decrease of hemoglobin in red blood cells, a condition known as iron-deficiency _____.

11. A CVA on the left side of the brain can cause a deficit or loss of speech, known as _____.

1. resection
2. prolapse
3. post mortem
4. tachycardia
5. neonatal
6. remission

7. transurethral
8. post partum
9. paralysis
10. anemia
11. aphasia

K. Circle the term that best completes the meaning of the sentences in the following medical vignettes:

1. As part of her (**intravenous, post partum, antenatal**) care, Bea underwent (**ultrasonography, endoscopy, urinalysis**) to determine the fetal age and to make sure that there were no anatomical anomalies.

2. Ellen's pregnancy test was positive but she had excruciating pelvic pain. After an examination and ultrasound, the doctors diagnosed a(an) (**epidural, ectopic, subscapular**) pregnancy. She then underwent emergency surgery to remove the early pregnancy from the fallopian tube.

3. After noticing a suspicious-looking mole on her upper arm, Carole was diagnosed with (**malignant, benign, subtotal**) melanoma. This type of skin cancer is a(an) (**intrauterine, extrahepatic, neoplastic**) process and has a high likelihood of (**paralysis, dysplasia, metastasis**) to other areas of the body.

4. Carole's daughter, Annabelle, found a mole on her back and quickly had it checked out by her physician. Fortunately, after a biopsy, the pathology revealed a (**transabdominal, precancerous, perianal**) nevus (mole) that was considered (**chronic, unilateral, benign**). In the future, Annabelle will need close follow-up for other suspicious lesions.

5. Milton's blood pressure was 160/110. Normal blood pressure is 120/80. Because of his (**bradycardia, hypertension, dyspnea**), Milton's physician prescribed medication to reduce his risk of stroke.

1. antenatal, ultrasonography
2. ectopic
3. malignant, neoplastic, metastasis
4. precancerous, benign
5. hypertension

V. REVIEW

Write the meaning of each of the following word parts. Please don't forget to check your answers with the answer keys at the end of this review section.

PREFIXES

PREFIX	MEANING	PREFIX	MEANING
1. a-, an-	_____	20. inter-	_____
2. ab-	_____	21. intra-	_____
3. ad-	_____	22. mal-	_____
4. ana-	_____	23. meta-	_____
5. ante-	_____	24. neo-	_____
6. anti-	_____	25. para-	_____
7. bi-	_____	26. peri-	_____
8. brady-	_____	27. post-	_____
9. con-	_____	28. pre-	_____
10. dia-	_____	29. pro-, pros-	_____
11. dys-	_____	30. quadri-	_____
12. ec-	_____	31. re-, retro-	_____
13. endo-	_____	32. sub-	_____
14. epi-	_____	33. syn-	_____
15. ex-, extra-	_____	34. tachy-	_____
16. hemi-	_____	35. trans-	_____
17. hyper-	_____	36. tri-	_____
18. hypo-	_____	37. ultra-	_____
19. in-	_____	38. uni-	_____

COMBINING FORMS

COMBINING FORM	MEANING	COMBINING FORM	MEANING
1. abdomin/o	_____	16. neur/o	_____
2. an/o	_____	17. norm/o	_____
3. bi/o	_____	18. oste/o	_____
4. cardi/o	_____	19. peritone/o	_____
5. carp/o	_____	20. plas/o	_____
6. cis/o	_____	21. ren/o	_____
7. cost/o	_____	22. scapul/o	_____
8. crani/o	_____	23. son/o	_____
9. cutane/o	_____	24. thyroid/o	_____
10. dur/o	_____	25. top/o	_____
11. gen/o	_____	26. troph/o	_____
12. glyc/o	_____	27. urethr/o	_____
13. hemat/o	_____	28. uter/o	_____
14. later/o	_____	29. ven/o	_____
15. nat/i	_____	30. vertebr/o	_____

SUFFIXES

SUFFIX	MEANING	SUFFIX	MEANING
1. -al	_____	4. -crine	_____
2. -ation	_____	5. -dipsia	_____
3. -cision	_____	6. -emia	_____

7. -gen _____

8. -graphy _____

9. -ia _____

10. -ic _____

11. -ine _____

12. -ism _____

13. -lysis _____

14. -mortem _____

15. -oma _____

16. -ous _____

17. -partum _____

18. -pathy _____

19. -plasm _____

20. -pnea _____

21. -rrhea _____

22. -scopy _____

23. -section _____

24. -stasis _____

25. -tension _____

26. -thesis _____

27. -tic _____

28. -um _____

29. -uria _____

30. -y _____

PREFIXES

◆ **ANSWER KEY**

1. no, not, without
2. away from
3. toward
4. up, apart
5. before, forward
6. against
7. two
8. slow
9. with, together
10. through, complete
11. bad, painful, difficult
12. out, outside
13. within, in, inner
14. above, upon
15. out, outside
16. half
17. excessive, above
18. below, under
19. in, into
20. between
21. within
22. bad
23. change, beyond
24. new
25. beside, near, along the side of
26. surrounding
27. after, behind
28. before
29. before, forward
30. four
31. back, behind
32. under, less than
33. with, together
34. fast
35. across, through
36. three
37. beyond
38. one

COMBINING FORMS

◆ **ANSWER KEY**

1. abdomen
2. anus
3. life
4. heart
5. wrist bones
6. to cut
7. ribs
8. skull
9. skin
10. dura mater
11. to produce
12. sugar
13. blood
14. side
15. birth
16. nerve
17. rule, order
18. bone
19. peritoneum
20. formation, growth
21. kidney
22. shoulder blade (bone)
23. sound
24. thyroid gland
25. to put, place
26. development, nourishment
27. urethra
28. uterus
29. vein
30. vertebra (backbone)

SUFFIXES

◆ **ANSWER KEY**

1. pertaining to
2. process, condition
3. process of cutting
4. secretion
5. condition of thirst
6. blood condition
7. to produce
8. process of recording
9. condition, process
10. pertaining to
11. pertaining to
12. condition, process
13. loosening, breakdown, separation, destruction
14. death
15. tumor
16. pertaining to
17. birth
18. disease condition
19. formation
20. breathing
21. flow, discharge
22. process of examining
23. incision
24. to stand, place, stop, control
25. pressure
26. to put, place
27. pertaining to
28. structure
29. urine condition
30. process, condition

VI. PRONUNCIATION OF TERMS

The terms that you have learned in this chapter are presented here with their pronunciations. The capitalized letters in boldface are the accented syllable. Pronounce each word out loud, then write its meaning in the space provided.

TERM	PRONUNCIATION	MEANING
abnormal	ab-**NOR**-mal	
adrenal glands	ah-**DRE**-nal glanz	
analysis	ah-**NAL**-ih-sis	
anemia	ah-**NE**-me-ah	
ante mortem	**AN**-te **MOR**-tem	
ante partum	**AN**-te **PAR**-tum	
ante natal	**AN**-te **NA**-tal	
antibiotic	an-tih-bi-**OT**-ik	
antibody	**AN**-tih-bod-e	
antigen	**AN**-tih-jen	
aphasia	a-**FA**-ze-ah	
apnea	**AP**-ne-ah	
atrophy	**AT**-ro-fe	
benign	be-**NIN**	
bilateral	bi-**LAT**-er-al	
bradycardia	bra-de-**KAR**-de-ah	
congenital anomaly	kon-**JEN**-ih-tal ah-**NOM**-ah-le	
dialysis	di-**AL**-ih-sis	

diarrhea	di-ah-**RE**-ah
dysphagia	dis-**FA**-jah
dysplasia	dis-**PLA**-zhah
dyspnea	**DISP**-ne-ah or disp-**NE**-ah
dysuria	dis-**U**-re-ah
ectopic pregnancy	ek-**TOP**-ik **PREG**-nan-se
endocrine glands	**EN**-do-krin glanz
endoscopy	en-**DOS**-ko-pe
epidural hematoma	ep-ih-**DUR**-al he-mah-**TO**-mah
excision	ek-**SIZH**-un
extrahepatic	eks-tra-heh-**PAT**-ik
hemigastrectomy	heh-me-gast-**REK**-to-me
hemiplegia	heh-me-**PLE**-jah
hyperglycemia	hi-per-gli-**SE**-me-ah
hypertension	hi-per-**TEN**-shun
hyperthyroidism	hi-per-**THI**-royd-izm
hypertrophy	hi-**PER**-tro-fe
hypoglycemia	hi-po-gli-**SE**-me-ah
incision	in-**SIZH**-un
intervertebral	in-ter-**VER**-teh-bral
intrauterine	in-trah-**U**-ter-in
intravenous	in-trah-**VE**-nus
malignant	mah-**LIG**-nant

metacarpal	met-ah-**KAR**-pal
metastasis	meh-**TAS**-tah-sis
neonatal	ne-o-**NA**-tal
neoplastic	ne-o-**PLAS**-tik
paralysis	pah-**RAL**-ih-sis
paraplegia	par-ah-**PLE**-jah
parathyroid glands	par-ah-**THI**-royd glanz
perianal	per-e-**A**-nal
periosteum	per-e-**OS**-te-um
polydipsia	pol-e-**DIP**-se-ah
polyneuropathy	pol-e-nu-**ROP**-ah-the
polyuria	pol-e-**UR**-e-ah
post mortem	post **MOR**-tem
post partum	post **PAR**-tum
precancerous	pre-**KAN**-ser-us
prolapse	pro-**LAPS**
prosthesis	pros-**THE**-sis
quadriplegia	quah-drah-**PLE**-jah
relapse	re-**LAPS**
remission	re-**MISH**-un
resection	re-**SEK**-shun
retroperitoneal	reh-tro-peri-ih-to-**NE**-al
subcostal	sub-**KOS**-tal

subcutaneous   sub-ku-**TA**-ne-us _____

subdural hematoma   sub-**DUR**-al he-mah-**TO**-mah _____

subscapular   sub-**SKAP**-u-lar _____

subtotal   sub-**TO**-tal _____

syndrome   **SIN**-drom _____

tachycardia   tak-eh-**KAR**-de-ah _____

tachypnea   tak-ip-**NE**-ah _____

transabdominal   trans-ab-**DOM**-ih-nal _____

transurethral   trans-u-**RE**-thral _____

tricuspid valve   tri-**KUS**-pid valv _____

ultrasonography   ul-trah-son-**OG**-rah-fe _____

unilateral   u-nih-**LAT**-er-al _____

urinalysis   u-rih-**NAL**-ih-sis _____

VII. PRACTICAL APPLICATIONS

A. Match the abnormal condition in Column I with the organ lesion or body part in Column II that may be the cause of the condition:

COLUMN I		COLUMN II
1. aphasia	_____	A. urinary bladder
2. dysphagia	_____	B. colon
3. diarrhea	_____	C. uterine cervix
4. quadriplegia	_____	D. left-sided brain lesion
5. hyperglycemia	_____	E. pancreas

6. dysuria	_____	F. lungs	
7. paraplegia	_____	G. heart	
8. bradycardia	_____	H. cervical spinal cord lesion	
9. dyspnea	_____	I. esophagus	
10. dysplasia	_____	J. lumbar spinal cord lesion	

◆ **ANSWER KEY**   1. D   2. I   3. B   4. H   5. E
6. A   7. J   8. G   9. F   10. C

B. Pathology: Disease description—HYPERTHYROIDISM
  From the following terms complete the sentences in the paragraphs below:

bradycardia	hypersecretion	hyposecretion	hypoplastic
dyspnea	antibodies	antibiotics	goiter
tachycardia	hyperplastic	exophthalmos	neoplastic

Hyperthyroidism, also known as thyrotoxicosis or Graves disease, is marked by

an excess of thyroid hormones. There is much evidence to support a hereditary factor

in the development of this condition and some consider it an autoimmune disorder

caused by _____ that bind to the surface of thyroid gland cells and

stimulate _____ of hormones (T_3 and T_4— triiodothyronine and

thyroxine). The enlarged gland, histologically, is composed of _____

follicles lined with hyperactive cells.

Symptoms of hyperthyroidism include restlessness, insomnia, weight loss,

sweating, and rapid heartbeat or _____. Abnormal protrusion of the

eyes, known as _____, is another symptom. The patient also has an

enlarged thyroid gland, called a _____.

◆ **ANSWER KEY**

antibodies	tachycardia
hypersecretion	exophthalmos
hyperplastic	goiter

CHAPTER 5

MEDICAL SPECIALISTS AND CASE REPORTS

CHAPTER SECTIONS

CHAPTER OBJECTIVES

- To describe the training process of physicians
- To identify medical specialists and describe their specialties
- To identify combining forms used in terms that describe specialists
- To decipher medical terminology as written in case reports

I. INTRODUCTION

This chapter reviews many of the terms you have learned in previous chapters while adding others related to medical specialists. In Section II, the training of physicians is described and specialists are listed with their specialties. Section III uses combining forms, which are found in the terms describing specialists, with familiar suffixes to test your knowledge of terms. In Section IV, short case reports are presented to illustrate the use of the medical language in context. As you read these reports, you will be impressed with your ability to understand medical terminology!

II. MEDICAL SPECIALISTS

Doctors complete four years of medical school then pass National Medical Board Examinations to receive an M.D. (Medical Doctor) degree. They may then begin post-graduate training, the length of which is at least three years and in some cases longer. This postgraduate training is known as *residency training*. Examples of residency programs are:

Anesthesiology	Administration of agents capable of bringing about a loss of sensation
Dermatology	Diagnosis and treatment of skin disorders
Emergency medicine	Care of patients that requires sudden and immediate action
Family practice	Primary care of all members of the family on a continuing basis
Internal medicine	Diagnosis of disorders and treatment with drugs
Ophthalmology	Diagnosis and treatment of eye disorders
Pathology	Diagnosis of the cause and nature of disease
Pediatrics	Diagnosis and treatment of children's disorders
Psychiatry	Diagnosis and treatment of disorders of the mind
Radiology	Diagnosis using x-rays and other procedures (ultrasound and magnetic resonance imaging)
Surgery	Treatment by manual (SURG- means "hand") or operative methods

Examinations are administered after the completion of each residency program to certify the doctor's competency in that specialty area.

A physician may then choose to specialize further by doing *fellowship training*. Fellowships (lasting two to five years) train doctors in *clinical* (patient care) and *research* (laboratory) skills. For example, an *internist* (specialist in internal medicine) may choose fellowship training in internal medicine specialties such as neurology, nephrology, endocrinology, and oncology. A surgeon interested in further specialization may do fellowship training in thoracic surgery, neurosurgery, or plastic surgery. On completion of training and examinations, the doctor is then recognized as a specialist in that specialty area.

Medical specialists and an explanation of their specialties are listed below:

MEDICAL SPECIALIST	SPECIALTY
allergist	Treatment of hypersensitivity reactions
anesthesiologist	Administration of agents for loss of sensation
cardiologist	Treatment of heart disease
cardiovascular surgeon	Surgery on the heart and blood vessels
colorectal surgeon	Surgery on the colon and rectum
dermatologist	Treatment of skin disorders
emergency practitioner	Immediate evaluation and treatment of people with acute injury and illness in a hospital setting
endocrinologist	Treatment of endocrine gland disorders
family practitioner	Primary care and treatment of families on a continuing basis
gastroenterologist	Treatment of stomach and intestinal disorders
geriatrician	Treatment of diseases of old age
gynecologist	Surgery and treatment of the female reproductive system
hematologist	Treatment of blood disorders
infectious disease specialist	Treatment of diseases caused by microorganisms
internist	Comprehensive care to adults in an office or hospital
nephrologist	Treatment of kidney diseases
neurologist	Treatment of nerve disorders
neurosurgeon	Surgery on the brain, spinal cord, and nerves
obstetrician	Treatment of pregnant women; delivery of babies
oncologist	Diagnosis and medical treatment of malignant and benign tumors
ophthalmologist	Surgical and medical treatment of eye disorders
orthopedist	Surgical treatment of bones, muscles, and joints
otolaryngologist	Treatment of the ear, nose, and throat
pathologist	Diagnosis of disease by analysis of cells
pediatrician	Treatment of diseases of children
physical medicine and rehabilitation specialist	Treatment to restore function after illness
psychiatrist	Treatment of mental disorders
pulmonary specialist	Treatment of lung diseases
radiologist	Examination of x-rays to determine a diagnosis; includes interpretation of ultrasound images and MRI and nuclear medicine as well
radiation oncologist	Treatment of disease with high-energy radiation
rheumatologist	Treatment of joint and muscle disorders
thoracic surgeon	Surgery on chest organs
urologist	Surgery on the urinary tract

III. COMBINING FORMS AND VOCABULARY

The combining forms listed below should be familiar because they are found in the list
of terms describing medical specialists. A medical term is included to illustrate the use
of the combining form. Write the meaning of the medical term in the space provided.
You can always check your answers with the glossary at the end of the book.

COMBINING FORM	MEANING	MEDICAL TERM	MEANING
cardi/o	heart	cardiomegaly	_____
col/o	colon	colostomy	_____
dermat/o	skin	dermatitis	_____
endocrin/o	endocrine glands	endocrinology	_____
enter/o	intestines	enteritis	_____
esthesi/o	sensation	anesthesiology	_____
gastr/o	stomach	gastroscopy	_____
ger/o	old age	geriatrics	_____
gynec/o	woman, female	gynecology	_____
hemat/o	blood	hematoma	_____
iatr/o	treatment	iatrogenic	_____
		IATR/O- means "treatment by a physician or with medicines." An iatrogenic illness is *produced* (-GENIC) unexpectedly by a treatment.	
laryng/o	voice box	laryngeal	_____
nephr/o	kidney	nephrostomy	_____
neur/o	nerve	neuralgia	_____

nos/o	disease	nosocomial _____
		A nosocomial infection is acquired during
		hospitalization (COMI/O- means "to care for").
obstetr/o	midwife	obstetric _____
onc/o	tumor	oncogenic _____
		Oncogenic viruses give rise to tumors.
ophthalm/o	eye	ophthalmologist _____
opt/o	eye	optometrist _____
		An optometrist examines (METR/O- means "to
		measure") eyes and prescribes glasses but cannot
		treat eye diseases.
		optician _____
		Opticians grind lenses and fit glasses but do not
		examine eyes, prescribe glasses, or treat eye
		diseases.
orth/o	straight	orthopedist _____
		PED/O- comes from the Greek, *paidos,* meaning
		"child." In the past, orthopedists were concerned
		with straightening bone deformities in children.
		Now, they treat bone, muscle, and joint disorders in
		adults as well.
ot/o	ear	otitis _____
path/o	disease	pathology _____
ped/o	child	pediatrics _____
psych/o	mind	psychosis _____
pulmon/o	lung	pulmonary _____
radi/o	x-rays	radiotherapy _____
		Radiotherapy is also called *radiation therapy.* See
		Figure 5-1.
rect/o	rectum	rectocele _____
		-CELE means "a hernia or protrusion." The walls of
		the rectum weaken and bulge forward toward the
		vagina. See Figure 5-2.

FIGURE 5-1

Radiation therapy. The patient is positioned under a radiation therapy machine (linear accelerator) to receive treatment for a lesion in the posterior portion of his hip. (Courtesy Dr. Arthur Brimberg, Riverhill Radiation Oncology, Yonkers, NY.)

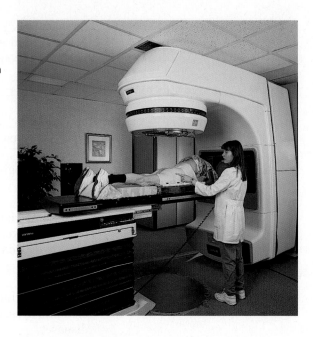

FIGURE 5-2

Rectocele. (Modified from Chabner D-E: *The Language of Medicine,* ed 6, Philadelphia, 2001, WB Saunders.)

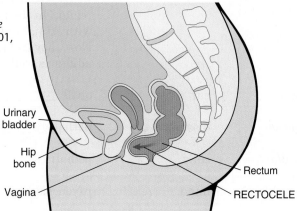

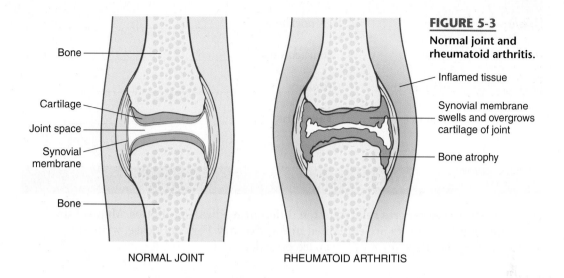

FIGURE 5-3

Normal joint and rheumatoid arthritis.

Bone

Cartilage

Joint space

Synovial membrane

Bone

NORMAL JOINT

Inflamed tissue

Synovial membrane swells and overgrows cartilage of joint

Bone atrophy

RHEUMATOID ARTHRITIS

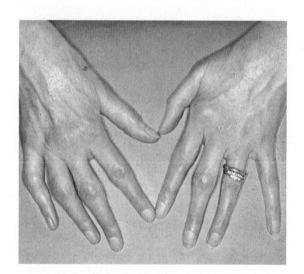

FIGURE 5-4

Advanced rheumatoid arthritis of the hands. (From *Mosby's Medical, Nursing, & Allied Health Dictionary,* ed 5, St Louis, 1998, Mosby.)

rheumat/o   flow, fluid

rheumatology _____

Joints can fill with fluid when diseased, hence RHEUMAT/O- indicates a problem with a swollen joint. Rheumatoid arthritis is a chronic inflammatory disease of joints and connective tissues that leads to deformation of joints. See Figures 5-3 and 5-4.

rhin/o	nose	rhinorrhea _____
thorac/o	chest	thoracotomy _____
ur/o	urinary tract	urology _____
vascul/o	blood vessels	vasculitis _____

IV. CASE REPORTS

Here are short case reports related to ten different medical specialties. Many of the terms are familiar; others are explained in the glossary. For every case, write the meaning of the boldface term in the space provided.

CASE 1 ◆ Cardiology

Mr. Rose was admitted to the Cardiac Care Unit (CCU) after a severe **myocardial infarction.** He had suffered from **angina** (due to **ischemia**), and **hypertension** for some time previously. He is being treated with **antiarrhythmic** drugs, **diuretics,** and **anticoagulants.** If his recovery proceeds as expected, he will be discharged in three weeks.

angina _____

antiarrhythmic _____

anticoagulant _____

diuretic _____

hypertension _____

ischemia _____

myocardial infarction _____

CASE 2 ◆ Gynecology

Ms. Sessions has been complaining of **dysmenorrhea** and **menorrhagia** for several months. She is also **anemic.** Because of the presence of large **fibroids,** as seen on a pelvic **ultrasound** exam (**sonogram**), a **hysterectomy** is recommended.

anemic _____

dysmenorrhea _____

fibroids _____

hysterectomy _____

menorrhagia _____

sonogram _____

ultrasound _____

CASE 3 ◆ Oncology

The patient is a 26-year-old female with a previous diagnosis of **mediastinal** and **intra-abdominal Hodgkin disease.** She was admitted to the hospital for **lymphangiography** and **percutaneous** liver **biopsy** after the discovery of possible recurrence of tumor. Following the assessment of her **platelet** count, a percutaneous liver biopsy was performed, showing normal **hepatic** tissue. The **lymphangiogram** was normal as well. The patient was later scheduled for **peritoneoscopy.**

biopsy _____

hepatic _____

Hodgkin disease _____

intra-abdominal _____

lymphangiogram _____

lymphangiography _____

mediastinal _____

percutaneous _____

peritoneoscopy _____

platelet _____

CASE 4 ◆ Urology

Polly Smith has a history of lower back pain associated with **hematuria** and **dysuria.** She has an appointment at the hospital for investigation of her symptoms. Tests include an **intravenous pyelogram** (IVP) and **cystoscopy.** The findings of these tests confirmed the diagnosis of **renal calculus. Lithotripsy** was recommended, and her **prognosis** is favorable.

calculus _____

cystoscopy _____

dysuria _____

hematuria _____

intravenous pyelogram (IVP) _____

lithotripsy _____

prognosis _____

renal _____

CASE 5 ◆ Gastroenterology

Mr. Pepper suffers from **dyspepsia** and sharp **abdominal** pain. A recent episode of **hematemesis** has left him very weak and **anemic. Gastroscopy** and **barium meal (swallow)** revealed the presence of a large **ulcer.** He will be admitted to the hospital and scheduled for a partial **gastrectomy.**

abdominal _____

anemic _____

barium meal (swallow) _____

dyspepsia _____

gastrectomy _____

gastroscopy _____

hematemesis _____

ulcer _____

CASE 6 ◆ Radiology

Examination: **Thoracic cavity.** PA **(posterior-anterior)** and **lateral** chest. There is a patchy **infiltrate** in the right lower **lobe** seen best in the lateral view. The heart and **mediastinal** structures are normal. No evidence of **pleural effusion.**
Impression: Right lower lobe **pneumonia**

anterior _____

infiltrate _____

lateral _____

lobe _____

mediastinal _____

pleural effusion _____

pneumonia _____

posterior _____

thoracic cavity _____

CASE 7 ◆ Orthopedics

A 20-year-old male patient was admitted to the hospital following a motorcycle accident. In the accident he sustained **fractures** of the right **tibia**, right **femur,** and **pelvis** and **intra-abdominal** injuries. Two pins were placed through the lower and upper end of the tibia, and a cast was applied. Two days later he was taken to surgery, and internal **fixation** of the right femur was performed.

femur _____

fixation _____

fracture _____

intra-abdominal _____

pelvis _____

tibia _____

CASE 8 ◆ Nephrology

A 52-year-old man with **chronic renal failure** secondary to long-standing **hypertension** has been maintained on **hemodialysis** for the past 18 months. For the past three weeks during the dialysis sessions he has become moderately **hypotensive,** with symptoms of dizziness. Consequently, we have decided to withhold his **antihypertensive** medications prior to dialysis.

antihypertensive _____

chronic _____

hemodialysis _____

hypertension _____

hypotensive _____

renal failure _____

CASE 9 ◆ Endocrinology

A 36-year-old woman known to have **insulin**-dependent **diabetes mellitus** (Type I) was brought to the emergency room after being found collapsed in her home. She had experienced three days of extreme weakness, **polyuria,** and **polydipsia.** It was discovered that a few days prior to her admission she had discontinued her insulin in a suicide attempt.

diabetes mellitus _____

insulin _____

polydipsia _____

polyuria _____

CASE 10 ◆ Neurology

Ms. Rose is admitted with severe, throbbing **unilateral frontal cephalgia** that has lasted for two days. Light makes her cringe and she complains of **nausea**. Before the onset of these symptoms, she saw zigzag lines for about 20 minutes. Diagnosis is **acute migraine** with **aura**. A **vasoconstrictor** is prescribed, and Ms. Rose's condition is improving. (Migraine headaches are thought to be caused by sudden **dilation** of blood vessels.)

acute _____

aura _____

cephalgia _____

dilation _____

frontal _____

migraine _____

nausea _____

unilateral _____

vasoconstrictor _____

V. EXERCISES AND ANSWERS

These exercises test your understanding of the terms in Sections II and III. Don't forget to check your responses with the answers directly following each exercise.

A. Match each of the following residency programs to its description below:

internal medicine	pediatrics	psychiatry
radiology	surgery	family practice
anesthesiology	emergency medicine	pathology
dermatology	ophthalmology	

1. Treatment by operation or manual (hand) methods: _____

2. Diagnosis of adult disorders and treatment with drugs: _____

3. Diagnosis and treatment of disorders of the mind: _____

4. Primary care of all family members on a continuing basis: _____

5. Diagnosis and treatment of skin disorders: _____

6. Diagnosis and treatment of eye disorders: _____

7. Diagnosis of disease using x-rays: _____

8. Diagnosis and treatment of children's disorders: _____

9. Care of patients that requires immediate action: _____

10. Administration of agents that cause loss of sensation: _____

11. Diagnosis of disease by examining cells and tissues: _____

◆ **ANSWER KEY**
1. surgery	7. radiology
2. internal medicine	8. pediatrics
3. psychiatry	9. emergency medicine
4. family practice	10. anesthesiology
5. dermatology	11. pathology
6. ophthalmology	

B. Name the doctor who treats the following problems (first letters are given):

1. Kidney diseases   N _____

2. Tumors   O _____

3. Broken bones   O _____

4. Female diseases   G _____

5. Eye disorders   O _____

6. Heart disorders   C _____

7. Nerve disorders   N _____

8. Lung disorders   P _____

9. Mental disorders   P _____

10. Stomach and intestinal disorders   G _____

◆ **ANSWER KEY**
1. nephrologist
2. oncologist
3. orthopedist
4. gynecologist
5. ophthalmologist
6. cardiologist (internist) or cardiovascular surgeon (surgeon)
7. neurologist
8. pulmonary specialist
9. psychiatrist
10. gastroenterologist

C. Match the medical specialists in Column I to their specialties in Column II:

COLUMN I

1. urologist   ____

2. thoracic surgeon   ____

3. radiation oncologist   ____

4. colorectal surgeon   ____

5. endocrinologist   ____

6. obstetrician   ____

7. radiologist   ____

8. pediatrician   ____

9. hematologist   ____

10. dermatologist   ____

COLUMN II

A. Operates on the large intestine

B. Treats blood disorders

C. Treats thyroid and pituitary gland disorders

D. Delivers babies

E. Treats children and their disorders

F. Operates on the urinary tract

G. Treats disorders of the skin

H. Treats tumors by using high-energy radiation

I. Operates on the chest

J. Examines x-rays to diagnose disease

◆ **ANSWER KEY**   1. F   2. I   3. H   4. A   5. C
                              6. D   7. J   8. E   9. B   10. G

D. Complete each of the sentences below using a term from the following list:

clinical	optician	surgeon
pathologist	oncologist	infectious disease specialist
ophthalmologist	optometrist	geriatrician
orthopedist	research	

1. A physician who diagnoses and treats diseases that are caused by microorganisms

   is a(an) _____.

2. A doctor who does bone surgery is a(an) _____.

3. A doctor who takes care of patients does _____ medicine.

4. A person who grinds lenses and fills prescriptions for eye glasses is a(an)

   _____.

5. A doctor who reads biopsy samples and performs autopsies is a(an)

   _____.

6. A doctor who treats cancerous tumors is a(an) _____.

7. A person who can examine eyes and prescribe eye glasses but cannot treat eye

   disorders is a(an) _____.

8. A doctor who operates on patients is a(an) _____.

9. A doctor who does experiments with test tubes and laboratory equipment is

   interested in _____ medicine.

10. A doctor who specializes in treatment of disorders of the eye is a(an)

    _____.

11. A doctor who specializes in the treatment of older people is a(an)

    _____.

◆ **ANSWER KEY**

1. infectious disease specialist	4. optician
2. orthopedist	5. pathologist
3. clinical	6. oncologist

7. optometrist	10. ophthalmologist
8. surgeon	11. geriatrician
9. research	

E. Which medical specialist would you consult for the following medical conditions? The first letter of the specialist is given.

1. Arthritis   R _____

2. Otitis media   O _____

3. Anemia   H _____

4. Urinary bladder displacement   U _____

5. Chronic bronchitis   P _____

6. Cerebrovascular accident   N _____

7. Breast cancer   O _____

8. Hole in the wall of the heart   C _____

9. Dislocated shoulder bone   O _____

10. Thyroid gland enlargement   E _____

11. Kidney disease   N _____

12. Acne (skin disorder)   D _____

13. Hay fever (hypersensitivity reaction)   A _____

14. Viral and bacterial diseases   I _____

◆ **ANSWER KEY**

1. rheumatologist	8. cardiovascular surgeon
2. otolaryngologist	9. orthopedist
3. hematologist	10. endocrinologist
4. urologist	11. nephrologist
5. pulmonary specialist	12. dermatologist
6. neurologist	13. allergist
7. oncologist	14. infectious disease specialist

F. Give the meaning for each of the following medical terms:

1. neuralgia _____

2. pathology _____

3. cardiomegaly _____

4. nephrostomy _____

5. thoracotomy _____

6. laryngeal _____

7. otitis _____

8. colostomy _____

9. pulmonary _____

10. iatrogenic _____

11. gastroscopy _____

12. radiotherapy _____

13. anesthesiology _____

14. enteritis _____

15. nosocomial _____

◆ **ANSWER KEY**
1. nerve pain
2. study of disease
3. enlargement of the heart
4. opening from the kidney to the outside of the body
5. incision of the chest
6. pertaining to the voice box
7. inflammation of the ear
8. opening of the colon to the outside of the body
9. pertaining to the lungs
10. pertaining to an abnormal condition that has been produced by treatment
11. process of visual examination of the stomach

12. treatment of disease using high-energy radiation
13. study of loss of sensation or feeling
14. inflammation of the intestines (usually small intestine)
15. pertaining to a disease acquired in the hospital

G. **Use the following combining forms and suffixes to make the medical terms called for:**

COMBINING FORMS		SUFFIXES	
laryng/o	nephr/o	-itis	-scopy
neur/o	ophthalm/o	-ectomy	-osis
onc/o	thorac/o	-tomy	-logy
col/o	ot/o	-algia	-therapy
psych/o	path/o	-genic	-stomy

1. Inflammation of the ear: _____

2. Removal of a nerve: _____

3. Incision of the chest: _____

4. Study of tumors: _____

5. Pertaining to producing disease: _____

6. Inflammation of the voice box: _____

7. Opening of the large intestine to the outside of the body: _____

8. Visual examination of the eye: _____

9. Abnormal condition of the mind: _____

10. Inflammation of the kidney: _____

11. Removal of the large intestine: _____

12. Pain in the ear: _____

13. Treatment of the mind: _____

14. Pertaining to producing tumors: _____

◆ **ANSWER KEY**

1. otitis
2. neurectomy
3. thoracotomy
4. oncology
5. pathogenic
6. laryngitis
7. colostomy
8. ophthalmoscopy
9. psychosis
10. nephritis
11. colectomy
12. otalgia
13. psychotherapy
14. oncogenic

H. Circle the term that best completes the meaning of the sentences in the following medical vignettes:

1. Dr. Butler is a specialized physician who operates on hearts. He trained as a **(neurologic, cardiovascular, pulmonary)** surgeon. Often, his procedures require that Dr. Smith, a(an) **(gynecologic, ophthalmic, thoracic)** surgeon, assist him when the chest and lungs need surgical intervention.

2. Pauline noticed a rash over most of her body. First she saw Dr. Cole, her **(family practitioner, oncologist, radiologist)** who performs her yearly physicals. Dr. Cole, who is not a(an) **(endocrinologist, orthopedist, dermatologist)** by training, referred her to a skin specialist to make the proper diagnosis and treat the rash.

3. Dr. Liu is a(an) **(internist, obstetrician, pediatrician)** as well as a(an) **(nephrologist, urologist, gynecologist,)** and can take care of her female patients before, during, and after their pregnancies.

4. After her sixth pregnancy, Sally developed an abnormal condition at the lower end of her colon. She went to a(an) **(gastroenterologist, hematologist, optometrist)**, who made the diagnosis of protrusion of the rectum into the vagina. She then consulted colorectal and gynecologic surgeons to make an appropriate treatment plan for her condition, known as a **(vasculitis, rectocele, colostomy)**.

5. In the cancer clinic, patients often must see a medical **(oncologist, orthopedist, rheumatologist)** who administers chemotherapy, and a(an) **(psychiatrist, radiation oncologist, radiologist)** who prescribes **(drugs, surgery, radiation therapy)** to treat tumors with high-energy protons and electrons.

6. While recovering from successful surgery in the hospital, Janet developed a cough and fever. Her surgeon ordered a chest x-ray and suspected a(an) **(oncogenic, nosocomial, iatrogenic)** pneumonia. A(an) **(anesthesiologist, neurologist, infectious disease specialist)** was called in to diagnose and treat the hospital-acquired disease condition.

1. cardiovascular, thoracic
2. family practitioner, dermatologist
3. obstetrician, gynecologist
4. gastroenterologist, rectocele
5. oncologist, radiation oncologist, radiation therapy
6. nosocomial, infectious disease specialist

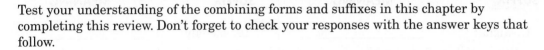

VI. REVIEW

Test your understanding of the combining forms and suffixes in this chapter by completing this review. Don't forget to check your responses with the answer keys that follow.

COMBINING FORMS

COMBINING FORM	MEANING	COMBINING FORM	MEANING
1. cardi/o		13. nephr/o	
2. col/o		14. neur/o	
3. dermat/o		15. nos/o	
4. endocrin/o		16. obstetr/o	
5. enter/o		17. onc/o	
6. esthesi/o		18. ophthalm/o	
7. gastr/o		19. opt/o	
8. ger/o		20. orth/o	
9. gynec/o		21. ot/o	
10. hemat/o		22. path/o	
11. iatr/o		23. ped/o	
12. laryng/o		24. psych/o	

25. pulmon/o _____

26. radi/o _____

27. rect/o _____

28. rheumat/o _____

29. rhin/o _____

30. thorac/o _____

31. ur/o _____

32. vascul/o _____

SUFFIXES

SUFFIX	MEANING	SUFFIX	MEANING
1. -algia	_____	9. -megaly	_____
2. -ary	_____	10. -oma	_____
3. -cele	_____	11. -osis	_____
4. -eal	_____	12. -rrhea	_____
5. -genic	_____	13. -scopy	_____
6. -ist	_____	14. -stomy	_____
7. -itis	_____	15. -therapy	_____
8. -logy	_____	16. -tomy	_____

COMBINING FORMS

◆ **ANSWER KEY**

1. heart
2. colon
3. skin
4. endocrine glands
5. intestines
6. sensation
7. stomach
8. old age
9. woman
10. blood
11. treatment
12. voice box
13. kidney
14. nerve
15. disease
16. midwife
17. tumor
18. eye
19. eye
20. straight
21. ear
22. disease
23. child
24. mind
25. lung
26. x-rays

27. rectum	30. chest
28. flow, fluid	31. urinary tract
29. nose	32. blood vessels

SUFFIXES

◆ **ANSWER KEY**

1. pain	10. mass, tumor
2. pertaining to	11. abnormal condition
3. hernia, protrusion	12. flow
4. pertaining to	13. process of visual
5. pertaining to producing	examination
6. specialist	14. opening
7. inflammation	15. treatment
8. study of	16. incision
9. enlargement	

VII. PRONUNCIATION OF TERMS

The terms that you have learned in this chapter are presented here with their pronunciations. The capitalized letters in boldface represent the accented syllable. Pronounce each word out loud, then write the meaning in the space provided.

TERM	PRONUNCIATION	MEANING
anesthesiology	an-es-the-ze-**OL**-o-je	
cardiologist	kar-de-**OL**-o-jist	
cardiovascular surgeon	kar-de-o-**VAS**-ku-lar **SUR**-jin	
clinical	**KLIN**-eh-kal	
colorectal surgeon	ko-lo-**REK**-tal **SUR**-jin	
colostomy	ko-**LOS**-to-me	
dermatologist	der-mah-**TOL**-o-jist	
dermatology	der-mah-**TOL**-o-je	
emergency medicine	e-**MER**-jen-se **MED**-ih-sin	

endocrinologist	en-do-krih-**NOL**-o-jist _____
enteritis	en-teh-**RI**-tis _____
family practitioner	**FAM**-ih-le prak-**TIH**-shan-er _____
gastroenterologist	gas-tro-en-ter-**OL**-o-jist _____
gastroscopy	gas-**TROS**-ko-pe _____
geriatric	jer-e-**AH**-trik _____
geriatrician	jer-e-ah-**TRISH**-shan _____
gynecologist	gi-neh-**KOL**-o-jist _____
gynecology	gi-neh-**KOL**-o-je _____
hematologist	he-mah-**TOL**-o-jist _____
hematoma	he-mah-**TO**-mah _____
iatrogenic	i-ah-tro-**JEN**-ik _____
infectious disease	in-**FEK**-shus dih-**ZEZ** _____
internal medicine	in-**TER**-nal **MED**-ih-sin _____
laryngitis	lah-rin-**JI**-tis _____
nephrologist	neh-**FROL**-o-jist _____
nephrostomy	neh-**FROS**-to-me _____
neuralgia	nu-**RAL**-jah _____
neurologist	nu-**ROL**-o-jist _____
neurosurgeon	nu-ro-**SUR**-jin _____
nosocomial	nos-o-**KO**-me-al _____
obstetrician	ob-steh-**TRISH**-un _____
obstetrics	ob-**STET**-riks _____

oncogenic	ong-ko-**JEN**-ik
oncologist	ong-**KOL**-o-jist
ophthalmologist	of-thal-**MOL**-o-jist
ophthalmology	of-thal-**MOL**-o-je
optician	op-**TISH**-an
optometrist	op-**TOM**-eh-trist
orthopedist	or-tho-**PE**-dist
otitis	o-**TI**-tis
otolaryngologist	o-to-lah-rin-**GOL**-o-jist
pathologist	pah-**THOL**-o-jist
pathology	pah-**THOL**-o-je
pediatric	pe-de-**AT**-rik
pediatrician	pe-de-ah-**TRISH**-un
psychiatrist	si-**KI**-ah-trist
psychosis	si-**KO**-sis
pulmonary specialist	**PUL**-mo-ner-e **SPESH**-ah-list
radiation oncologist	ra-de-**A**-shun ong-**KOL**-o-jist
radiologist	ra-de-**OL**-o-jist
radiotherapy	ra-de-o-**THER**-ah-pe
rectocele	**REK**-to-sel
research	**RE**-surch
rheumatologist	roo-mah-**TOL**-o-jist
rheumatology	roo-mah-**TOL**-o-je

rhinorrhea	ri-no-**RE**-ah _____
surgery	**SUR**-jer-e _____
thoracic surgeon	tho-**RAS**-ik **SUR**-jin _____
thoracotomy	tho-rah-**KOT**-o-me _____
urologist	u-**ROL**-o-jist _____
vasculitis	vas-ku-**LI**-tis _____

VIII. PRACTICAL APPLICATIONS

The exercises in this section are divided into three groups, each of which consists of a list of allied health specialists followed by a set of job descriptions. For each group, match each specialist to the appropriate job description and then check your answers with the answer key at the end of the Practical Applications section.

Group A

1. nurse anesthetist _____

2. audiologist _____

3. blood bank technologist _____

4. chiropractor _____

5. clinical laboratory technician _____

6. dental assistant _____

7. dental hygienist _____

8. dental laboratory technician _____

9. diagnostic medical sonographer _____

10. dietitian/nutritionist _____

a) Treats patients with health problems associated with the muscular, nervous, and skeletal systems, especially the spine
b) Prepares materials (crowns, bridges) for use by a dentist

c) Works with people who have hearing problems by using testing devices to measure hearing loss
d) Provides preventive dental care and teaches the practice of good oral hygiene
e) Collects, types, and prepares blood and its components for transfusions
f) Aids in the delivery of anesthesia during surgery
g) Assists a dentist with dental procedures
h) Performs diagnostic ultrasound procedures
i) Plans nutrition programs and supervises the preparation and serving of meals
j) Performs tests to examine and analyze body fluids, tissues, and cells

Group B

1. EKG technician _____

2. emergency medical technician/paramedic _____

3. health information management professional _____

4. home health aide _____

5. licensed practical nurse _____

6. medical assistant _____

7. medical laboratory technician _____

8. nuclear medicine technologist _____

9. nursing aide _____

10. occupational therapist _____

a) Cares for elderly, disabled, and ill persons in their own homes, helping them live there instead of in an institution
b) Performs routine tests and laboratory procedures
c) Designs, manages, and administers the use of heath care data and information
d) Operates an electrocardiograph to record EKGs, Holter monitoring, and stress tests
e) Performs radioactive tests and procedures under the supervision of a nuclear medicine physician, who interprets the results
f) Gives immediate care and transports sick or injured to medical facilities
g) Helps physicians examine and treat patients and performs tasks to keep offices running smoothly
h) Cares for the sick, injured, convalescing, and handicapped, under the direct supervision of physicians and registered nurses; provides basic bedside care

i) Helps individuals with mentally, physically, developmentally, emotionally disabling conditions to develop, recover, or maintain daily living and working skills

j) Helps care for physically or mentally ill, injured, or disabled patients confined to nursing, hospital, or residential care facilities; known as nursing assistants or hospital attendants

Group C

1. ophthalmic medical technician _____

2. phlebotomist _____

3. physical therapist _____

4. physician assistant _____

5. radiation therapist _____

6. radiographer/image technologist _____

7. registered nurse _____

8. respiratory therapist _____

9. speech language pathologist _____

10. surgical technologist _____

a) Evaluates, treats, and cares for patients with breathing disorders

b) Draws and tests blood under the supervision of a medical technologist or laboratory manager

c) Cares for sick and injured people by assessing and recording symptoms, assisting physicians during treatments and examinations, and administering medications

d) Prepares cancer patients for treatment and administers prescribed doses of ionizing radiation to specific areas of the body

e) Helps ophthalmologists provide medical eye care

f) Examines, diagnoses, and treats patients, under the direct supervision of a physician

g) Assists in operations under the supervision of surgeons or registered nurses

h) Improves the mobility, relieves the pain, and prevents or limits permanent physical disabilities of patients suffering from injuries or disease

i) Produces x-ray images of parts of the body for use in diagnosing medical problems

j) Assesses and treats persons with speech, language, voice, and fluency disorders

◆ ANSWER KEY

Group A

1. f	2. c	3. e	4. a	5. j
6. g	7. d	8. b	9. h	10. i

Group B

1. d	2. f	3. c	4. a	5. h
6. g	7. b	8. e	9. j	10. i

Group C

1. e	2. b	3. h	4. f	5. d
6. i	7. c	8. a	9. j	10. g

BODY SYSTEMS

This appendix contains full-color diagrams of body systems. Major organs and structures are labeled for your reference, and definitions for these parts on the body are listed in the Glossary of Medical Terms on p. 265. Combining forms for parts of the body are given in parentheses next to each label on the diagram. For easy reference, these combining forms are also listed in the Glossary of Word Parts on p. 299. This information will help you analyze medical terms as you work through the text.

On the page after each body systems diagram, you will find a list of combining forms and examples of terminology using each word part. This page also contains explanations of pathological conditions commonly associated with that body system. After this are selected descriptions of laboratory tests as well as diagnostic and treatment procedures for the body system. This appendix is organized as both a study tool for class and as a reference for your work in the medical field.

Circulation of Blood

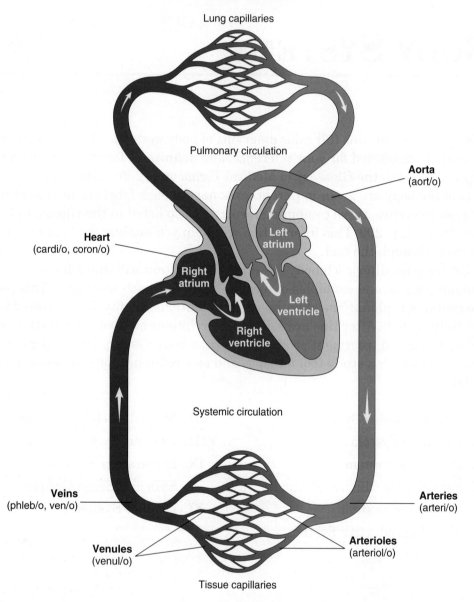

Red vessels contain blood that is rich in oxygen. Arrows show the path of blood flow from the tissue capillaries through venules and veins toward the heart, to the lung capillaries, back to the heart, out the aorta to the arteries and arterioles, and then back to the tissue capillaries.

TERMINOLOGY

Meanings for terminology are found in the Glossary of Medical Terms.

COMBINING FORM	MEANING	TERMINOLOGY	MEANING
angi/o	vessel	angioplasty _____	
aort/o	aorta	aortic stenosis _____	
arteri/o	artery	arteriosclerosis _____	
arteriol/o	arteriole	arteriolitis _____	
cardi/o	heart	cardiomyopathy _____	
coron/o	heart	coronary arteries _____	
phleb/o	vein	phlebotomy _____	
ven/o	vein	intravenous _____	
venul/o	venule	venulitis _____	

PATHOLOGY

Definitions for additional terms in boldface are found in the *Glossary of Medical Terms.*

Angina pectoris: Chest pain caused by decreased blood flow to heart muscle.

Aneurysm: Local widening of an artery caused by weakness in the arterial wall or breakdown of the wall owing to **atherosclerosis.**

Arrhythmia: Abnormal heart beat (rhythm); **fibrillation** and **flutter** are examples.

Atherosclerosis: Hardening of arteries with a collection of cholesterol-like plaque.

Congestive heart failure: Inability of the heart to pump its required amount of blood. Blood accumulates in the lungs, causing **pulmonary edema.**

Hypertension: High blood pressure. Essential hypertension is high blood pressure with no apparent cause. In secondary hypertension, another illness (kidney disease or an adrenal gland disorder) is the cause of the high blood pressure.

Myocardial infarction: Heart attack. An **infarction** is an area of dead **(necrotic)** tissue.

Shock: A group of symptoms (paleness of skin, weak and rapid pulse, shallow breathing) indicating poor oxygen supply to tissues and insufficient return of blood to the heart.

181

I. CARDIOVASCULAR SYSTEM—cont'd

LABORATORY TESTS

Lipid tests: Measurements of cholesterol and triglyceride levels in the blood.

Lipoprotein tests: Measurements of **high-density lipoprotein (HDL)** and **low-density lipoprotein (LDL)** in the blood.

Serum enzyme tests: Measurements of enzymes released into the bloodstream after a heart attack (myocardial infarction).

DIAGNOSTIC PROCEDURES

Angiography: Process of recording (via x-ray images) blood vessels after the injection of contrast into the bloodstream.

Cardiac catheterization: Process of introducing a catheter (a flexible, tubular instrument) into a vein or artery to measure pressure and flow patterns of blood.

Doppler ultrasound: Process of measuring blood flow in vessels via sound waves.

Echocardiography: Process of producing images of the heart via sound waves or echoes.

Electrocardiography: Process of recording electricity flowing through the heart.

Holter monitoring: Process of detecting abnormal heart rhythms **(arrhythmias)** that involves having a patient wear a compact version of an electrocardiograph for 24 hours.

Magnetic resonance imaging (MRI): Process of producing an image, by beaming magnetic waves at the heart, that gives detailed information about congenital heart disease, cardiac masses, and disease within large blood vessels.

MUGA scan: Process of imaging the motion of heart wall muscles and assessing the function of the heart via a *mu*ltiple-*g*ated *a*cquisition scan, which uses radioactive chemicals.

Positron emission tomography (PET scan): Process of injecting radioactive chemicals, which release radioactive particles that travel to the heart, to view cross-sectional images showing the flow of blood and the functional activity of the heart muscle.

Stress test: An electrocardiogram plus blood pressure and heart rate measurements that show the heart's response to physical exertion (treadmill test).

Thallium-201 scintigraphy: A radioactive test that shows where thallium-201 (a radioactive substance) localizes in heart muscle. Used with an exercise tolerance test (ETT), it detects heart muscle function. **Sestamibi,** or **ETT-MIBI,** scans are also used to detect blood perfusion in heart muscle.

Cardioversion: Brief discharges of electricity passing across the chest to stop a cardiac **arrhythmia.** Also called **defibrillation.**

Coronary artery bypass surgery (CABG): Procedure in which vessels taken from a patient's legs or chest are connected to coronary arteries to make detours around blockages.

Endarterectomy: Surgical removal of the innermost lining of an artery to remove fatty deposits and clots.

Heart transplantation: Procedure in which a donor heart is transferred to a recipient.

Percutaneous transluminal coronary angioplasty (PTCA): Procedure in which a balloon-tipped catheter (a flexible, tubular instrument) is threaded into a coronary artery to compress fatty deposits and open the artery. Stents (expandable slotted tubes) create wider openings that make the recurrence of blockages less likely.

Thrombolytic therapy: Procedure in which drugs, such as tPA (tissue plasminogen activator) and streptokinase, are injected into a patient's bloodstream to dissolve clots that may cause a heart attack.

ANATOMY

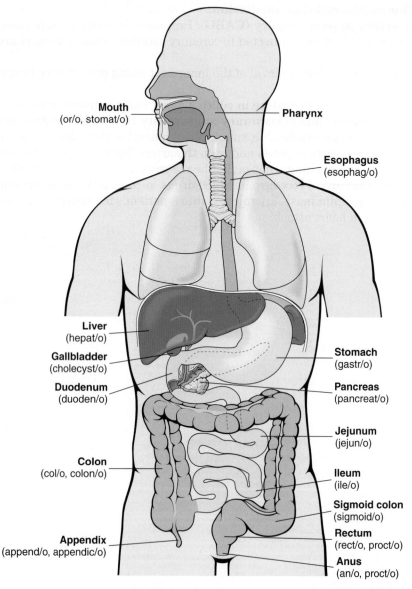

Mouth
(or/o, stomat/o)

Pharynx

Esophagus
(esophag/o)

Liver
(hepat/o)

Gallbladder
(cholecyst/o)

Duodenum
(duoden/o)

Stomach
(gastr/o)

Pancreas
(pancreat/o)

Jejunum
(jejun/o)

Colon
(col/o, colon/o)

Ileum
(ile/o)

Sigmoid colon
(sigmoid/o)

Appendix
(append/o, appendic/o)

Rectum
(rect/o, proct/o)

Anus
(an/o, proct/o)

Food enters the body via the mouth and travels through the pharynx, esophagus, and stomach to the small intestine (duodenum). The liver, gallbladder, and pancreas make and store chemicals that aid in the digestion of foods. Digested (broken down) food is absorbed into the bloodstream through the walls of the small intestine (jejunum and ileum). Any food that cannot be absorbed continues into the colon (large intestine) and leaves the body through the rectum and anus. (Adapted from Chabner D-E: *The Language of Medicine,* ed 6, Philadelphia, 2001, WB Saunders.)

TERMINOLOGY

COMBINING FORM	MEANING	TERMINOLOGY	MEANING
cholecyst/o	gallbladder	cholecystectomy _____	
col/o colon/o	colon	colostomy _____	
		colonoscopy _____	
duoden/o	duodenum	duodenal _____	
esophag/o	esophagus	esophageal _____	
gastr/o	stomach	gastralgia _____	
hepat/o	liver	hepatomegaly _____	
ile/o	ileum	ileostomy _____	
jejun/o	jejunum	gastrojejunostomy _____	
or/o	mouth	oral _____	
pancreat/o	pancreas	pancreatitis _____	
pharyng/o	pharynx	pharyngeal _____	
proct/o	anus and rectum	proctoscopy _____	
stomat/o	mouth	stomatitis _____	

PATHOLOGY

Cholelithiasis: Abnormal condition of gallstones.
Cirrhosis: Chronic disease of the liver with degeneration of liver cells.
Colonic polyposis: Condition in which **polyps** protrude from the mucous membrane lining the colon.
Diverticulosis: Abnormal condition of small pouches or sacs **(diverticula)** in the wall of the intestine (often the colon).
Gastroesophageal reflux disease (GERD): Backflow of the contents of the stomach into the esophagus.
Hepatitis: Inflammation of the liver.
Inflammatory bowel disease: Inflammation of the terminal (last) portion of the ileum **(Crohn disease)** or inflammation of the colon **(ulcerative colitis).**
Jaundice: Yellow-orange coloration of the skin and other tissues.

LABORATORY TESTS

Liver function tests (LFTs): Measurements of liver enzymes and other substances in the blood. Enzyme levels increase when the liver is damaged (as in hepatitis). Examples of liver enzymes are **ALT (SGPT), AST (SGOT),** and **alkaline phosphatase (alk phos).** High **bilirubin** (blood pigment) levels indicate **jaundice** caused by liver disease or other problems affecting the liver.

DIAGNOSTIC PROCEDURES

Abdominal computed tomography (CT scan): A series of cross-sectional x-ray images that show abdominal organs.
Abdominal magnetic resonance imaging (MRI): Process in which magnetic and radio waves create images of abdominal organs and tissues in all three planes of the body.
Abdominal ultrasound: Process of beaming sound waves into the abdomen to produce images of organs such as the gallbladder.
Barium tests: X-ray examinations using a liquid barium mixture to locate disorders of the gastrointestinal tract. In a **barium enema (lower GI series),** barium is injected into the anus and rectum and x-ray pictures are taken of the colon. In a **barium meal** or **swallow (upper GI series),** barium is swallowed and x-ray pictures are taken of the esophagus, stomach, and small intestine.

Cholangiography: X-ray examination of the bile ducts (CHOLANGI/O-) after the injection of contrast material through the liver (**percutaneous transhepatic cholangiography**) or through a catheter (a flexible, tubular instrument) from the mouth, esophagus, and stomach into the bile ducts (**endoscopic retrograde cholangiopancreatography** or **ERCP**).

Gastrointestinal endoscopy: Visual examination of the gastrointestinal tract using an endoscope. Examples are **esophagoscopy, gastroscopy,** and **sigmoidoscopy.**

Hemoccult test: A procedure in which feces is placed on paper containing the chemical guaiac, which reacts with hidden (occult) blood. This is an important screening test for colon cancer.

Stool culture: Feces (stools) are placed in a growth medium (culture) to test for microorganisms (such as bacteria).

TREATMENT PROCEDURES

Anastomosis: Surgical creation of an opening between two gastrointestinal organs. Examples are gastrojejunostomy, cholecystojejunostomy, and choledochoduodenostomy (CHOLEDOCH/O- means "common bile duct").

Colostomy: Surgical creation of a new opening of the colon to the outside of the body.

Ileostomy: Surgical creation of a new opening of the ileum to the outside of the body.

Laparoscopic surgery: Removal of organs and tissues via a laparoscope (instrument inserted into the abdomen through a small incision). Examples are **laparoscopic cholecystectomy** and **laparoscopic appendectomy.** Also known as **minimally invasive surgery.**

ANATOMY

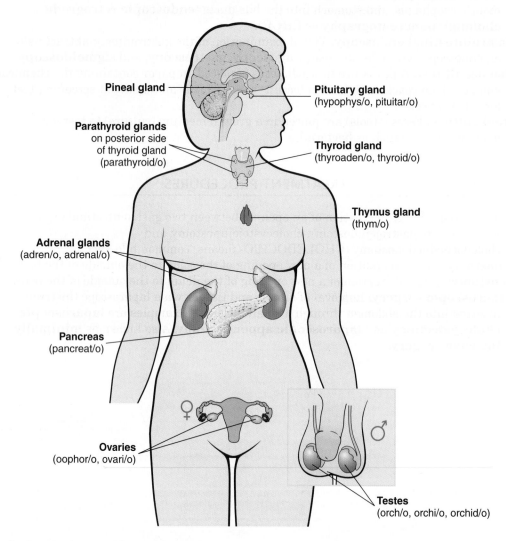

Pineal gland

Pituitary gland
(hypophys/o, pituitar/o)

Parathyroid glands
on posterior side
of thyroid gland
(parathyroid/o)

Thyroid gland
(thyroaden/o, thyroid/o)

Thymus gland
(thym/o)

Adrenal glands
(adren/o, adrenal/o)

Pancreas
(pancreat/o)

Ovaries
(oophor/o, ovari/o)

Testes
(orch/o, orchi/o, orchid/o)

Endocrine glands secrete (form and give off) hormones into the bloodstream. The hormones travel throughout the body, affecting organs (including other endocrine glands) and controlling their actions. (Modified from Chabner D-E: *The Language of Medicine,* ed 6, Philadelphia, 2001, WB Saunders.)

TERMINOLOGY

COMBINING FORM	MEANING	TERMINOLOGY	MEANING
adren/o adrenal/o	adrenal gland	adrenopathy _____	
		adrenalectomy _____	
hypophys/o	pituitary gland	hypophyseal _____	
oophor/o ovari/o	ovary	oophoritis _____	
		ovarian cyst _____	
orch/o orchi/o orchid/o	testis	orchitis _____	
		orchiopexy _____	
		orchidectomy _____	
pancreat/o	pancreas	pancreatectomy _____	
parathyroid/o	parathyroid gland	hyperparathyroidism _____	
pituitar/o	pituitary gland	hypopituitarism _____	
thym/o	thymus gland	thymoma _____	
thyroaden/o thyroid/o	thyroid gland	thyroadenitis _____	
		thyroidectomy _____	

PATHOLOGY

Acromegaly: Enlargement of extremities caused by hypersecretion from the anterior portion of the pituitary gland after puberty.

Cushing syndrome: A group of symptoms produced by excess secretion of **cortisol** from the adrenal cortex. These symptoms include obesity, moon-like fullness of the face, **hyperglycemia,** and **osteoporosis.**

Diabetes mellitus: A disorder of the pancreas that causes an increase in blood glucose levels. **Type 1 diabetes,** with the onset usually in childhood, involves complete deficiency of **insulin** in the body. **Type 2 diabetes,** with the onset usually in adulthood, involves some insulin deficiency and resistance of tissues to the action of insulin.

Goiter: Enlargement of the thyroid gland.

Hyperthyroidism: Overactivity of the thyroid gland; also called **Graves disease** or **exophthalmic** (eyeballs bulge outward) **goiter.**

LABORATORY TESTS

Fasting blood sugar: Measurement of glucose levels in a blood sample taken from a fasting patient and in specimens taken 30 minutes, 1 hour, 2 hours, and 3 hours after the ingestion of 75 gm of glucose. Delayed return of blood glucose to normal levels indicates **diabetes mellitus.**

Serum and urine tests: Measurement of hormones, **electrolytes,** and glucose levels in blood (serum) and urine as indicators of endocrine function.

Thyroid function tests: Measurement of levels of T_4 (thyroxine), T_3 (triiodothyronine), and TSH (thyroid-stimulating hormone) in the bloodstream.

Computed tomography (CT scan): Cross-sectional x-ray images of the pituitary gland and other endocrine organs.

Exophthalmometry: Measurement of eyeball protrusion **(exophthalmos)** as an indicator of **Graves disease (hyperthyroidism).**

Radioactive iodine uptake: The uptake of radioactive iodine, given by mouth, measured as evidence of thyroid function.

Thyroid scan: Procedure in which a radioactive compound, injected intravenously, localizes in the thyroid gland. A scanning device produces an image showing the presence of tumors or nodules in the gland.

ANATOMY

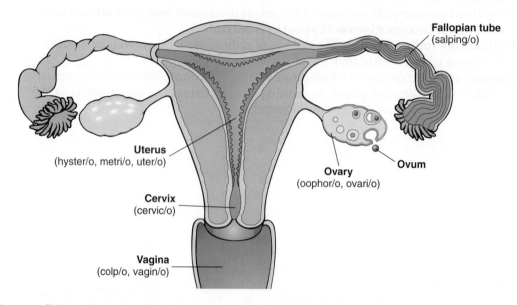

Fallopian tube
(salping/o)

Uterus
(hyster/o, metri/o, uter/o)

Ovary
(oophor/o, ovari/o)

Ovum

Cervix
(cervic/o)

Vagina
(colp/o, vagin/o)

An egg cell (ovum) is produced in the ovary and travels through the fallopian tube. If a sperm cell is present and fertilization (the union of the egg and sperm cell) takes place, the resulting cell (embryo) may implant in the lining of the uterus. The embryo (later called the fetus) develops in the uterus for nine months and is delivered from the body through the cervix and vagina. (Modified from Chabner D-E: *The Language of Medicine,* ed 6, Philadelphia, 2001, WB Saunders.)

TERMINOLOGY

COMBINING FORM	MEANING	TERMINOLOGY	MEANING
cervic/o	cervix	cervical _____	
colp/o vagin/o	vagina	colposcopy _____	
		vaginitis _____	
hyster/o metri/o uter/o	uterus	hysterectomy _____	
		endometrium _____	
		uterine _____	
oophor/o ovari/o	ovary	oophorectomy _____	
		ovarian cancer _____	
salping/o	fallopian tube	salpingectomy _____	

PATHOLOGY

Amenorrhea: Absence of menstrual flow.

Dysmenorrhea: Painful menstrual flow.

Ectopic pregnancy: Pregnancy that is not in the uterus; usually occurring in a fallopian tube.

Endometriosis: Tissue from the inner lining of the uterus (**endometrium**) occurs abnormally in other pelvic or abdominal locations (**fallopian tubes, ovaries,** or **peritoneum**).

Fibroids: Benign tumors in the uterus. Also called a **leiomyoma;** LEI/O- means "smooth."

Menorrhagia: Excessive discharge (-RRHAGIA) of blood from the uterus during **menstruation.**

Pelvic inflammatory disease: Inflammation (often caused by bacterial infection) in the region of the pelvis. Because the condition primarily affects the fallopian tubes, it is also called **salpingitis.**

LABORATORY TEST

Pregnancy test: Measurement of human chorionic gonadotropin (HCG), a hormone in blood and urine that indicates pregnancy.

DIAGNOSTIC PROCEDURES

Aspiration: Withdrawal of fluid from a cavity or sac. In breast aspiration, a needle is used to remove fluid from cystic lesions in the breast. The fluid is analyzed for the presence of malignant cells.

Colposcopy: Visual examination of the vagina and cervix using a colposcope (a small, magnifying instrument resembling a mounted pair of binoculars).

Conization: Removal of a cone-shaped section of the cervix for **biopsy.**

Hysterosalpingography: X-ray imaging of the uterus and fallopian tubes after injection of a contrast material into the uterus.

Mammography: X-ray imaging of the breast.

Pap smear: Procedure in which a physician inserts a wooden spatula or cotton swab to take secretions from the cervix and vagina. Microscopic analysis of the smear (spread on a glass slide) indicates the presence of cervical or vaginal disease.

Pelvic ultrasonography: Procedure that produces an image of sound waves as they bounce off organs (such as the ovaries and uterus) in the pelvic (hip) region. In **transvaginal ultrasound,** a sound probe is placed in the vagina.

Cauterization: The use of heat to destroy abnormal tissue, such as can occur, for example, in the lining of the **cervix** (lower neck-like region of the uterus).

Cryosurgery: The use of cold temperatures (liquid nitrogen) to freeze and destroy tissue (such as the lining of the cervix).

Dilation and curettage (D&C): Widening (dilation) of the opening of the cervix and scraping (curettage) of the lining of the uterus to remove tissue and stop prolonged or heavy uterine bleeding.

Myomectomy: The removal of **fibroid (myoma)** tissue from the uterus.

Tubal ligation: Procedure in which both fallopian tubes are ligated (tied off) in two places with sutures and the intervening segment is burnt or removed. This prevents pregnancy.

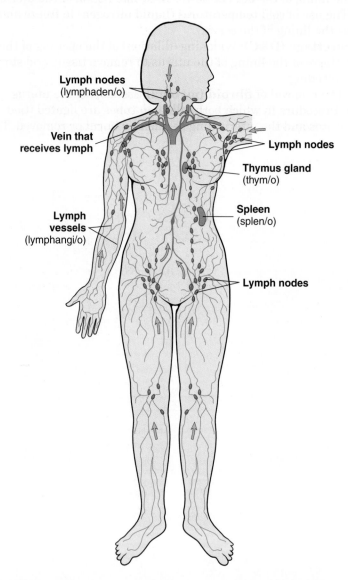

Lymph nodes
(lymphaden/o)

Vein that receives lymph

Lymph nodes

Thymus gland
(thym/o)

Spleen
(splen/o)

Lymph vessels
(lymphangi/o)

Lymph nodes

Lymph originates in the tissue spaces around cells and travels in lymph vessels and through lymph nodes to a large vein in the neck, where it enters the bloodstream. Lymph contains white blood cells (lymphocytes) that help the body fight disease. The spleen produces lymphocytes and disposes of dying blood cells. The thymus gland also produces lymphocytes. (Modified from Chabner D-E: *The Language of Medicine,* ed 6, Philadelphia, 2001, WB Saunders.)

COMBINING FORM	MEANING	TERMINOLOGY	MEANING
lymph/o	lymph fluid	lymphoma _____	
lymphaden/o	lymph node ("gland")	lymphadenectomy _____	
		lymphadenopathy _____	
lymphangi/o	lymph vessel	lymphangiography _____	
splen/o	spleen	splenomegaly _____	
thym/o	thymus gland	thymoma _____	

PATHOLOGY

Acquired immunodeficiency syndrome (AIDS): Suppression or deficiency of the immune response (destruction of **lymphocytes**) caused by exposure to **human immunodeficiency virus (HIV).**

Lymphoma: Malignant tumor of lymph nodes and lymphatic tissue. **Hodgkin disease** is an example of a lymphoma.

Mononucleosis: Acute infectious disease with enlargement of lymph nodes and increased numbers of **lymphocytes** and **monocytes** in the bloodstream.

Sarcoidosis: Inflammatory disease in which small nodules, or tubercles, form in lymph nodes and other organs. SARC/O- means "flesh," and -OID means "resembling."

LABORATORY TESTS

ELISA (*en*zyme-*l*inked *i*mmuno*s*orbent *a*ssay): A test to screen for antibodies to the **human immunodeficiency virus,** which causes **acquired immunodeficiency syndrome (AIDS).**

Western blot test: A blood test to detect the presence of antibodies to specific antigens such as the **human immunodeficiency virus (HIV).** It is regarded as a more precise test than the ELISA.

DIAGNOSTIC PROCEDURES

Computed tomography (CT scan): X-ray views in the transverse plane for the diagnosis of abnormalities in lymphoid organs (lymph nodes, spleen, and thymus gland).

Lymphangiography: X-ray imaging of lymph nodes and vessels after the injection of contrast into the lymphatic system in the soft tissue of the foot.

Chemotherapy: Treatment with powerful drugs to kill cancer cells (**Hodgkin disease,** non-Hodgkin lymphoma, and multiple myeloma) and viruses such as the **human immunodeficiency virus.**

Radiotherapy (radiation therapy): Treatment with high-dose radiation to destroy malignant lesions in the body.

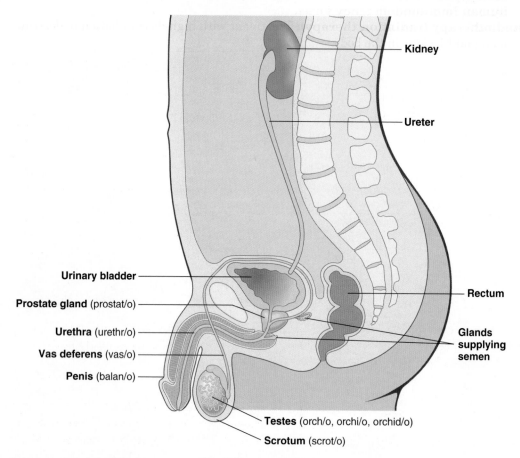

Kidney

Ureter

Urinary bladder

Prostate gland (prostat/o)

Urethra (urethr/o)

Vas deferens (vas/o)

Penis (balan/o)

Rectum

Glands supplying semen

Testes (orch/o, orchi/o, orchid/o)

Scrotum (scrot/o)

Sperm cells are produced in the testes (singular: testis) and travel up into the body, through the vas deferens, and around the urinary bladder. The vas deferens unites with the urethra, which opens to the outside of the body through the penis. The prostate and the other glands near the urethra produce a fluid (semen) that leaves the body with sperm cells.

TERMINOLOGY

COMBINING FORM	MEANING	TERMINOLOGY	MEANING
balan/o	penis	balanitis _____	
orch/o orchi/o orchid/o	testis	orchitis _____ orchiectomy _____ orchidectomy _____	
prostat/o	prostate gland	prostatectomy _____	
scrot/o	scrotum	scrotal _____	
urethr/o	urethra	urethritis _____	
vas/o	vas deferens	vasectomy _____	

PATHOLOGY

Benign prostatic hyperplasia: Noncancerous enlargement of the prostate gland.
Cryptorchism: Condition of undescended testis. The testis is not in the scrotal sac at birth. CRYPT/O- means "hidden."
Hydrocele: Sac of clear fluid in the scrotum. HYDR/O- means "water," and -CELE indicates a hernia (a bulging or swelling).
Prostatic carcinoma: Cancer of the prostate gland.
Testicular carcinoma: Malignant tumor of the testis. An example is a **seminoma.**
Varicocele: Enlarged, swollen veins near a testicle. VARIC/O- means "swollen veins."

LABORATORY TESTS

Protein-specific antigen (PSA): Measurement of the amount of PSA in the blood. Higher than normal levels are associated with prostatic enlargement and prostate cancer.

Semen analysis: Measurement of the number, shape, and motility (ability to move) of sperm cells.

DIAGNOSTIC PROCEDURE

Digital rectal examination (DRE): Examination of the prostate gland using finger palpation through the rectum.

TREATMENT PROCEDURES

Orchiopexy: Surgical fixation (-PEXY) of an undescended testicle in a young male infant.

Transurethral resection of the prostate gland (TURP): The removal of portions of the prostate gland using an **endoscope** inserted into the urethra.

Vasectomy: Procedure in which the vas deferens on each side is cut, a piece is removed, and the free ends are folded and ligated (tied) with sutures. Vasectomy produces sterilization so that sperm are not released with semen.

ANATOMY

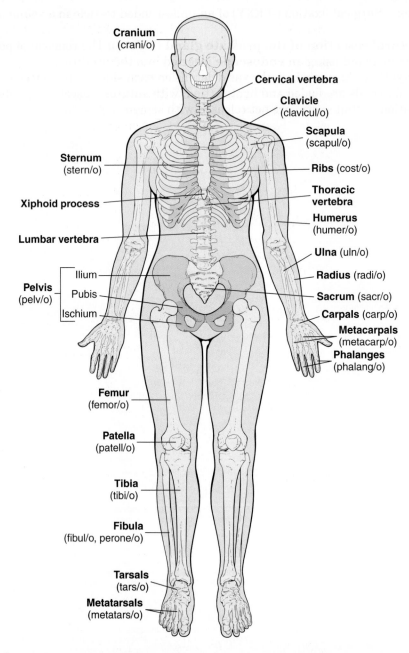

Cranium
(crani/o)

Cervical vertebra

Clavicle
(clavicul/o)

Scapula
(scapul/o)

Sternum
(stern/o)

Ribs (cost/o)

Thoracic
vertebra

Xiphoid process

Humerus
(humer/o)

Lumbar vertebra

Ulna (uln/o)

Radius (radi/o)

Ilium

Pelvis
(pelv/o)

Pubis

Sacrum (sacr/o)

Ischium

Carpals (carp/o)

Metacarpals
(metacarp/o)

Phalanges
(phalang/o)

Femur
(femor/o)

Patella
(patell/o)

Tibia
(tibi/o)

Fibula
(fibul/o, perone/o)

Tarsals
(tars/o)

Metatarsals
(metatars/o)

Bones are connected to muscles that contract to move the body. Joints are the spaces between bones. Near the joints are ligaments that connect bones to other bones and tendons that connect bones to muscles. (Modified from Chabner D-E: *The Language of Medicine,* ed 6, Philadelphia, 2001, WB Saunders.)

TERMINOLOGY

COMBINING FORM	MEANING	TERMINOLOGY	MEANING
arthr/o	joint	arthroscopy _____	
chondr/o	cartilage	chondroma _____	
cost/o	rib	costochondritis _____	
crani/o	skull	craniotomy _____	
ligament/o	ligament	ligamentous _____	
my/o myos/o muscul/o	muscle	myosarcoma _____	
		myositis _____	
		muscular _____	
myel/o	bone marrow	myelodysplasia _____	
oste/o	bone	osteomyelitis _____	
pelv/o	pelvis, hipbone	pelvic _____	
spondyl/o vertebr/o	vertebra	spondylosis _____	
		intervertebral _____	
ten/o tendin/o	tendon	tenorrhaphy _____	
		tendinitis _____	

PATHOLOGY

Ankylosing spondylitis: Chronic, progressive **arthritis** with stiffening **(ankylosis)** of joints, primarily of the spine and hip.

Carpal tunnel syndrome: Compression of the median nerve as it passes between the ligament and the bones and tendons of the wrist.

Gouty arthritis: Inflammation of joints caused by excessive uric acid. Also called **gout.**

Muscular dystrophy: An inherited disorder characterized by progressive weakness and degeneration of muscle fibers.

Osteoporosis: Decrease in bone density with thinning and weakening of bone. -POROSIS means "containing passages or spaces."

Rheumatoid arthritis: Chronic inflammation of joints; pain, swelling, and stiffening, especially in the small joints of the hands and feet. RHEUM- means a "flowing," descriptive of the swelling in joints.

LABORATORY TESTS

Antinuclear antibody test (ANA): Test in which a sample of plasma is tested for the presence of antibodies found in patients with systemic lupus erythematosus.

Erythrocyte sedimentation rate (ESR): Measurement of the rate at which red blood cells fall to the bottom of a test tube. High sedimentation rates are associated with inflammatory diseases such as **rheumatoid arthritis.**

Serum calcium: Measurement of the amount of calcium in a sample of blood (serum). This test is important in evaluating diseases of bone.

Uric acid test: Measurement of the amount of uric acid in a sample of blood. High uric acid levels are associated with gouty arthritis.

DIAGNOSTIC PROCEDURES

Arthrocentesis: Surgical puncture to remove fluid from a joint.

Arthrography: X-ray imaging of a joint.

Arthroscopy: Visual examination of a joint using an arthroscope.

Bone scan: Procedure in which a radioactive substance is injected intravenously and its uptake in bones is measured using a special scanning device.

Electromyography (EMG): Recording of the strength of muscle contraction as a result of electrical stimulation.

Muscle biopsy: The removal of muscle tissue for microscopic examination.

TREATMENT PROCEDURES

Arthroplasty: Surgical repair of a joint. Total hip arthroplasty is the replacement of the head of the femur (thigh bone) and acetabulum (cup-shaped portion of the hip socket) with artificial parts **(prostheses)** that are cemented into the bone.

Chemonucleolysis: Treatment of a herniated disc by injection of chymopapain to dissolve the inner portion (nucleus) of the disc.

Endoscopic discectomy: Surgical removal of a herniated intervertebral disc using an endoscope.

Laminectomy: Surgical removal of a portion of a vertebra to allow visualization and removal of a portion of a protruding disc.

Microscopic discectomy: Surgical removal of a herniated intervertebral disc using an incision that is one to two inches long and visualization of the surgical field with an operating microscope.

ANATOMY

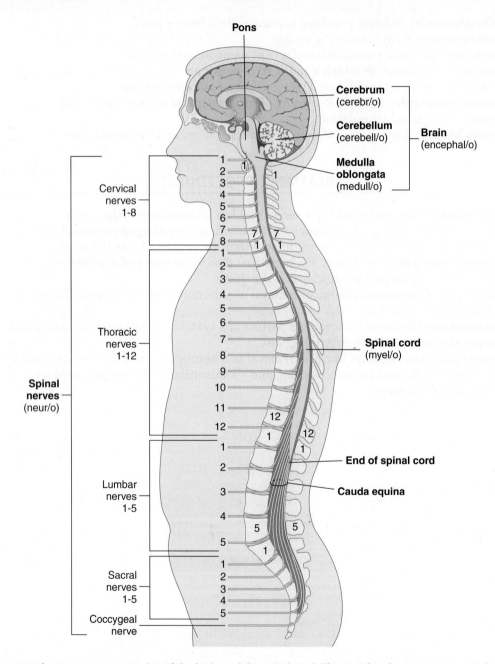

Pons

Cerebrum
(cerebr/o)

Cerebellum
(cerebell/o)

Brain
(encephal/o)

Medulla
oblongata
(medull/o)

Cervical
nerves
1-8

Thoracic
nerves
1-12

Spinal
nerves
(neur/o)

Spinal cord
(myel/o)

Lumbar
nerves
1-5

End of spinal cord

Cauda equina

Sacral
nerves
1-5

Coccygeal
nerve

The central nervous system consists of the brain and the spinal cord. The peripheral nervous system includes the nerves that carry messages to and from the brain and spinal cord. Spinal nerves carry messages to and from the spinal cord, and the cranial nerves (not pictured) carry messages to and from the brain.

TERMINOLOGY

COMBINING FORM	MEANING	TERMINOLOGY	MEANING
cerebell/o	cerebellum	cerebellar _____	
cerebr/o	cerebrum	cerebral _____	
encephal/o	brain	encephalitis _____	
medull/o	medulla oblongata	medullary _____	
myel/o	spinal cord	myelography _____	
neur/o	nerve	neuropathy _____	

PATHOLOGY

Alzheimer disease: Brain disorder marked by deterioration of mental capacity **(dementia).**

Cerebrovascular accident: Damage to the blood vessels of the cerebrum, leading to loss of blood supply to brain tissue; a **stroke.**

Concussion: Brief loss of consciousness as a result of injury to the brain.

Epilepsy: Chronic brain disorder characterized by recurrent **seizure** activity.

Glioblastoma: Malignant brain tumor arising from **neuroglial cells.** BLAST- means "immature."

Hemiplegia: Paralysis (-PLEGIA) that affects the right or left half of the body.

Meningitis: Inflammation of the **meninges** (membranes surrounding the brain and spinal cord).

Multiple sclerosis: Destruction of the **myelin sheath** on nerve cells in the central nervous system (brain and spinal cord), with replacement by plaques of sclerotic (hard) tissue.

Paraplegia: Paralysis that affects the lower portion of the body. From the Greek meaning "to strike" (-PLEGIA) on one side (PARA-). This term was previously used to describe **hemiplegia.**

Syncope: Fainting; sudden and temporary loss of consciousness as a result of inadequate flow of blood to the brain.

LABORATORY TEST

Cerebrospinal fluid (CSF) analysis: Chemical tests (for sodium, chloride, protein, and glucose), cell counts, cultures, and bacterial smears on samples of CSF to detect diseases of the brain or meninges. A lumbar puncture is used to remove CSF for analysis.

DIAGNOSTIC PROCEDURES

Cerebral angiography: Procedure in which x-ray films are taken of the blood vessels in the brain after the injection of contrast material into an artery.

Computed tomography (CT scan): Cross-sectional x-ray images of the brain and spinal cord (with and without contrast).

Electroencephalography (EEG): The recording of the electrical activity within the brain.

Lumbar puncture (LP): Procedure in which the pressure of CSF is measured and contrast may be injected for imaging **(myelography)** after removal of CSF from a space between the lumbar vertebrae. An LP or a spinal tap also provides a sample of cerebrospinal fluid for analysis.

Magnetic resonance imaging (MRI): Procedure in which magnetic waves and radiofrequency waves are used to create an image of the brain and spinal cord.

Myelography: X-ray imaging of the spinal cord after the injection of contrast.

Positron emission tomography (PET scan): Procedure in which the uptake of radioactive material in the brain shows how the brain uses glucose and gives information about brain function.

Stereotactic radiosurgery: Placement of the skull of a stereotactic instrument that locates a target (such as a tumor) in the brain. Then a high-energy radiation beam (gamma knife) is delivered to that precise target to destroy the tissue.

Transcutaneous electrical nerve stimulation (TENS): A battery-powered device delivers stimulation to nerves to relieve acute and chronic pain.

ANATOMY

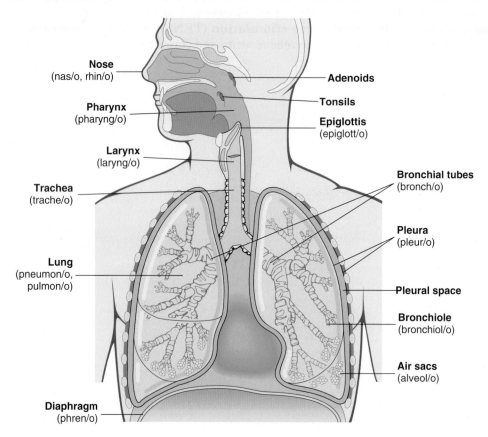

Nose
(nas/o, rhin/o)

Adenoids

Tonsils

Pharynx
(pharyng/o)

Epiglottis
(epiglott/o)

Larynx
(laryng/o)

Bronchial tubes
(bronch/o)

Trachea
(trache/o)

Pleura
(pleur/o)

Lung
(pneumon/o,
pulmon/o)

Pleural space

Bronchiole
(bronchiol/o)

Air sacs
(alveol/o)

Diaphragm
(phren/o)

Air enters the nose and travels to the pharynx (throat). From the pharynx, air passes through the epiglottis and larynx (voice box) into the trachea (windpipe). The trachea splits into two tubes, the bronchial tubes, that carry air into the lungs. The bronchial tubes divide into smaller tubes called bronchioles that end in small air sacs. Thin air sacs allow oxygen to pass through them into tiny capillaries containing red blood cells. Red blood cells transport the oxygen to all parts of the body. In a similar manner, gaseous waste (carbon dioxide) leaves the blood by entering air sacs and traveling out of the body through bronchioles, bronchial tubes, trachea, larynx, pharynx, and the nose.

TERMINOLOGY

COMBINING FORM	MEANING	TERMINOLOGY	MEANING
alveol/o	air sac; alveolus	alveolar _____	
bronch/o	bronchial tube	bronchoscopy _____	
bronchiol/o	bronchiole	bronchiolitis _____	
cyan/o	blue	cyanosis _____	
epiglott/o	epiglottis	epiglottitis _____	
laryng/o	larynx	laryngeal _____	
nas/o rhin/o	nose	nasal _____	
		rhinorrhea _____	
pharyng/o	pharynx	pharyngitis _____	
phren/o	diaphragm	phrenic _____	
pneumon/o pulmon/o	lung	pneumonectomy _____	
		pulmonary _____	
trache/o	trachea	tracheostomy _____	

PATHOLOGY

Asphyxia: Extreme decrease in the amount of **oxygen** in the body with increase of **carbon dioxide** leads to loss of consciousness or death.

Asthma: Spasm and narrowing of bronchi, leading to bronchial airway obstruction.

Atelectasis: Collapsed lung (ATEL/O- means "incomplete," and -ECTASIS indicates dilation or expansion).

Emphysema: Hyperinflation of air sacs with destruction of alveolar walls. Along with chronic **bronchitis** and **asthma,** emphysema is a type of **chronic obstructive pulmonary disease.**

Hemoptysis: Spitting up of blood.

Hemothorax: Blood in the pleural cavity (space between the **pleura**).

Pneumoconiosis: Abnormal condition of dust (CONI/O-) in the lungs.

Pneumonia: Inflammation and infection of alveoli, which fill with pus or products of the inflammatory reaction.

Tuberculosis: An infectious disease caused by bacteria (bacilli). The lungs and other organs are affected. Symptoms are cough, weight loss, night sweats, **hemoptysis,** and pleuritic pain.

LABORATORY TEST

Sputum analysis: Procedure in which a patient expels sputum by coughing, and the sputum is analyzed for bacterial content.

DIAGNOSTIC PROCEDURES

Bronchoscopy: Visual examination of the bronchial tubes using an endoscope.

Chest x-ray film: X-ray image of the chest in the A/P (antero-posterior), P/A (postero-anterior), and lateral (side) views.

Computed tomography (CT scan): Cross-sectional x-ray images of the chest.

Laryngoscopy: Visual examination of the larynx via the placement of a flexible tube (laryngoscope) through the nose or mouth and into the larynx.

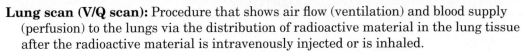

Lung scan (V/Q scan): Procedure that shows air flow (ventilation) and blood supply (perfusion) to the lungs via the distribution of radioactive material in the lung tissue after the radioactive material is intravenously injected or is inhaled.

Magnetic resonance imaging (MRI): Procedure in which magnetic waves and radiofrequency waves are used to create images of the chest in three planes of the body.

Pulmonary angiography: Procedure in which x-ray images are taken of the blood vessels in the lung after the injection of contrast material into a blood vessel. A blockage, such as a pulmonary embolism, can be located using this procedure.

Pulmonary function tests (PFTs): Measurement of the ventilation (breathing capability) of the lungs (air movement in and out of the lungs). A spirometer measures the air taken in and out of the lungs.

Tuberculin tests: Procedure in which agents are applied to the skin with punctures or injection and the reaction is noted. Redness and swelling result in people sensitive to the test substance and indicate prior or present infection with **tuberculosis.**

TREATMENT PROCEDURES

Endotracheal intubation: Procedure in which a tube is placed through the nose or mouth into the trachea to establish an airway during surgery and for placement on a respirator (a machine that moves air in and out of the lungs).

Thoracentesis: Procedure in which a needle is inserted through the skin between the ribs and into the pleural space to drain a **pleural effusion.**

Thoracotomy: Incision of the chest to remove a lung **(pneumonectomy)** or a portion of a lung (lobectomy).

Tracheostomy: Creation of an opening into the trachea through the neck and the insertion of a tube to create an airway.

ANATOMY

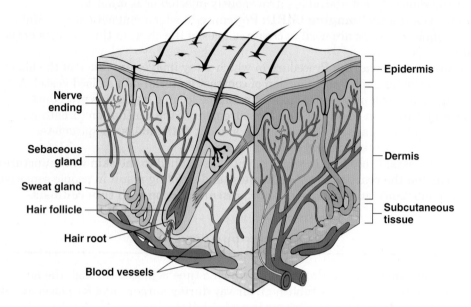

Skin (derm/o, dermat/o, cutane/o)

Epidermis

Nerve ending

Sebaceous gland

Sweat gland

Hair follicle

Hair root

Blood vessels

Dermis

Subcutaneous tissue

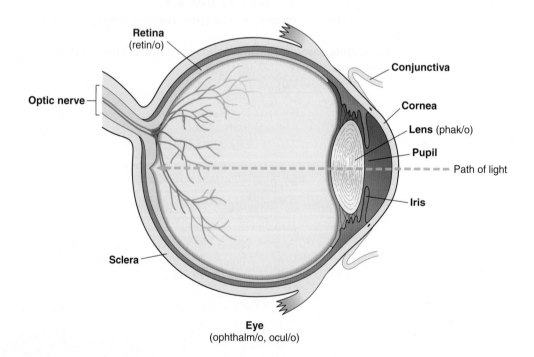

Eye
(ophthalm/o, ocul/o)

Retina (retin/o)

Optic nerve

Sclera

Conjunctiva

Cornea

Lens (phak/o)

Pupil

Path of light

Iris

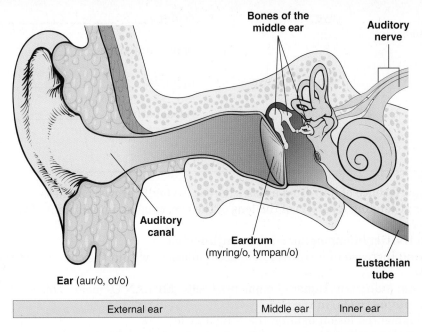

Bones of the middle ear

Auditory nerve

Auditory canal

Eardrum
(myring/o, tympan/o)

Eustachian tube

Ear (aur/o, ot/o)

| External ear | Middle ear | Inner ear |

The skin and sense organs receive messages (touch sensations, light waves, sound waves) from the environment and send them to the brain via nerves. These messages are interpreted in the brain, making sight, hearing, and perception of the environment possible. (Modified from Chabner D-E: *The Language of Medicine,* ed 6, Philadelphia, 2001, WB Saunders.)

TERMINOLOGY

COMBINING FORM	MEANING	TERMINOLOGY	MEANING
aur/o ot/o	ear	aural discharge _____	
		otitis _____	
cutane/o derm/o dermat/o	skin	subcutaneous _____	
		epidermis _____	
		dermatology _____	
myring/o tympan/o	eardrum	myringotomy _____	
		tympanoplasty _____	

ocul/o	eye	ocular _____
ophthalm/o		
		ophthalmoscope _____
phak/o	lens of the eye	aphakia _____
retin/o	retina	retinopathy _____

PATHOLOGY

Alopecia: Absence of hair from areas where it normally grows; baldness.
Cataract: Clouding (opacity) of the lens of the eye, causing impairment of vision or blindness.
Conjunctivitis: Inflammation of the **conjunctiva.**
Glaucoma: Increase in pressure (fluid accumulation) within the chamber at the front of the eye.
Melanoma: Malignant tumor of pigmented cells (MELAN/O- means "black") that arises from a **nevus** (mole) in the skin.
Nevus: Pigmented lesion in or on the skin; a mole.
Tinnitus: Abnormal noise (ringing, buzzing, roaring) sound in the ears.

LABORATORY TESTS

Bacterial and fungal tests: Procedures in which samples from skin lesions are taken to determine the presence of bacterial infection or fungal growth.

Fluorescein angiography: Procedure in which fluorescein (a dye) is injected intravenously and the movement of blood is observed by ophthalmoscopy. It is used to detect diabetic or hypertensive retinopathy and also degeneration of the macular (central) area of the retina.

Ophthalmoscopy: Visual examination of the interior of the eye.

Otoscopy: Visual examination of the eye (to the eardrum).

Skin biopsy: Procedure in which skin lesions are removed and sent to the pathology laboratory for microscopic examination.

Skin testing for allergy: Procedure in which allergy-causing substances are placed on the skin and a reaction is noted. In the patch test, a patch with a suspected allergen is placed on the skin. The scratch test involves making several scratches and the insertion of a small amount of allergen in the scratches.

Slit-lamp ocular examination: Procedure in which the anterior eye structures (such as the cornea) are microscopically examined using an instrument called a slit lamp.

Tuning fork tests: Procedure in which a vibration source (tuning fork) is placed in front of the opening to the ear to test air conduction of sound waves. The tuning fork is also placed on the mastoid bone behind the ear to test bone conduction of sound waves.

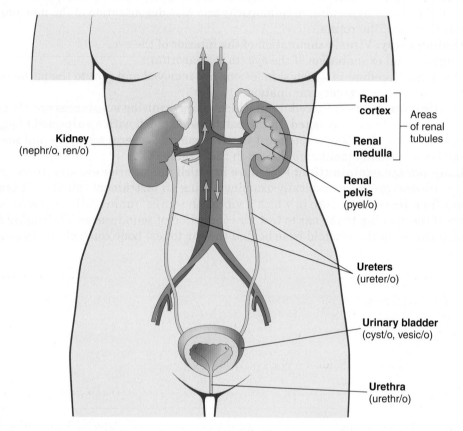

Kidney
(nephr/o, ren/o)

Renal cortex
Renal medulla
Areas of renal tubules

Renal pelvis
(pyel/o)

Ureters
(ureter/o)

Urinary bladder
(cyst/o, vesic/o)

Urethra
(urethr/o)

Urine is formed as waste materials, such as urea, are filtered from the blood into the tubules of the kidney. Urine passes from the tubules into the central collecting section of the kidney, the renal pelvis. Each renal pelvis leads directly to a ureter, which takes the urine to the urinary bladder. The bladder releases urine to the urethra and urine leaves the body.

COMBINING FORM	MEANING	TERMINOLOGY	MEANING
cyst/o vesic/o	urinary bladder	cystoscopy _____	
		vesical _____	
nephr/o ren/o	kidney	nephritis _____	
		renal _____	
pyel/o	renal pelvis	pyelogram _____	
ureter/o	ureter	ureterectomy _____	
urethr/o	urethra	urethritis _____	

PATHOLOGY

Albuminuria: Abnormal condition of protein (albumin) in the urine.
Anuria: Abnormal condition of no urine production.
Dysuria: Painful urination.
Glycosuria: Abnormal condition of glucose in the urine.
Hematuria: Abnormal condition of blood in the urine.
Nephrolithiasis: Abnormal condition of stones in the kidney.
Renal failure: Condition in which the kidneys stop functioning and do not produce urine.
Uremia: Condition of high levels of **urea** (nitrogenous waste material) in the blood.

LABORATORY TESTS

Blood urea nitrogen (BUN): Measurement of the amount of **urea** (nitrogenous waste) in the blood.

DIAGNOSTIC PROCEDURES

Cystoscopy: Visual examination of the urinary bladder using a **cystoscope** (endoscope).

Kidneys, ureters, bladder (KUB): X-ray image of the kidneys and urinary tract without the use of contrast.

Intravenous pyelogram (IVP): Procedure in which contrast material is injected intravenously and x-ray images are taken of the urinary tract (kidneys, ureters, bladder, and urethra).

Retrograde pyelogram (RP): Procedure in which contrast material is injected via a catheter (a flexible, tubular instrument) into the urethra and bladder and x-ray films are taken of the urethra, bladder, and ureters.

Voiding cystourethrogram (VCUG): Procedure in which x-ray films of the bladder and urethra are taken after the bladder is filled with a contrast material and while a patient is expelling urine.

Dialysis: Procedure in which waste materials (**urea, creatinine,** and uric acid) are separated from the blood by a machine **(hemodialysis).** Alternatively, a peritoneal catheter (a flexible, tubular instrument) delivers a special fluid into the abdominal cavity, and then a fluid, which contains waste materials that have seeped from the blood into it, is drained **(peritoneal dialysis).**

Extracorporeal shock wave lithotripsy (ESWL): Procedure in which shock waves are beamed into a patient to crush urinary tract stones. The stone fragments then pass out of the body with urine.

Renal transplantation: Procedure in which a donor kidney is transferred to a recipient.

Urinary catheterization: Procedure in which a catheter (a flexible, tubular instrument) is passed through the urethra and the urinary bladder for short- or long-term drainage of urine.

Major Classes of Drugs

Examples of drugs in each class are given by the lowercase **generic name** (official, nonproprietary) and then in uppercase and parentheses by the **trademark name** (chosen by the manufacturer).

ANALGESICS

Agents for the relief of pain

MILD

acetaminophen (Tylenol)
aspirin

NARCOTIC

codeine
hydromorphone (Dilaudid)
meperidine HCl (Demerol)
morphine sulfate
oxycodone HCl (OxyContin, Percodan)
propoxyphene (Darvon)

NSAIDS (NONSTEROIDAL ANTI-INFLAMMATORY DRUGS)

celecoxib (Celebrex)
diclofenac sodium (Arthrotec, Voltaren)
etodolac (Lodine)
ibuprofen (Motrin, Advil)
oxaprozin (Daypro)

ANESTHETICS

Agents for the reduction or elimination of sensation

GENERAL

ether
halothane (Fluothane)
midazolam HCl (Versed)
nitrous oxide
thiopental (Pentothal)

LOCAL

ethyl chloride
lidocaine HCl (Xylocaine)
procaine (Novocaine)

ANTIBIOTICS, ANTIFUNGALS, ANTITUBERCULARS, AND ANTIVIRALS

Agents for the inhibition or destruction of bacteria, fungi, parasites, and viruses

ANTIFUNGALS

amphotericin B (Fungizone)
fluconazole (Diflucan)
miconazole (Monistat)
nystatin (Nilstat)
terbinafine HCl (Lamisil)

ANTITUBERCULARS

isoniazid or INH (Nydrazid)
rifampin (Rifadin)

ANTIVIRALS

acyclovir (Zovirax)
indinavir (Crixivan)
lamivudine (Epivir)
zidovudine or AZT (Retrovir)

CEPHALOSPORINS: BACTERICIDAL AND SIMILAR TO PENICILLINS

cefprozil (Cefzil)
cefuroxime axetil (Ceftin)
cephalexin

ERYTHROMYCINS: BACTERIOSTATIC

azithromycin (Zithromax)
clarithromycin (Biaxin)
erythromycin (Ery-Tab)

PENICILLINS: BACTERICIDAL

amoxicillin trihydrate (Amoxil, Trimox)
amoxicillin with clavulanate (Augmentin)

QUINOLONES: BACTERICIDAL AND WIDE-SPECTRUM

ciprofloxacin (Cipro)
ofloxacin (Floxin)

SULFONAMIDES OR SULFA DRUGS: BACTERICIDAL

nitrofurantoin macrocrystals (Macrobid)
sulfamethoxazole with trimethoprim (Bactrim, Sulfatrim)
sulfisoxazole (Gantrisin)

TETRACYCLINES: BACTERICIDAL

doxycycline
tetracycline

ANTICOAGULANTS

Agents for the prevention of clotting

dicumarol
heparin
warfarin sodium (Coumadin)

ANTICONVULSANTS

Agents for the prevention or reduction of convulsions

clonazepam
divalproex sodium (Depakote)
gabapentin (Neurontin)
lorazepam (Ativan)
phenobarbital
phenytoin (Dilantin)

ANTIDEPRESSANTS

Agents for the treatment of symptoms of depression

amitriptyline HCl (Elavil)
bupropion (Wellbutrin SR)
citalopram hydrobromide (Celexa)
fluoxetine HCl (Prozac)
nefazodone HCl (Serzone)
venlafaxine (Effexor-XR)
paroxetine HCl (Paxil)
sertraline (Zoloft)

ANTIDIABETICS

Agents for the treatment of type 1 and type 2 diabetes

INSULINS

rDNA human insulin N (Humulin N)
rDNA human insulin lispro (Humalog)

ORAL DRUGS

acarbose (Precose)
glipizide (Glucotrol XL)
glyburide
glimepiride (Amaryl)
metformin (Glucophage)
repaglinide (Prandin)
troglitazone (Rezulin)

ANTIHISTAMINES

Agents that block the action of histamine, which is released in allergic reactions

cetirizine (Zyrtec)
dimenhydrinate (Dramamine)
diphenhydramine (Benadryl)
fexofenadine (Allegra)
loratadine (Claritin)

CARDIOVASCULAR DRUGS

Agents that act on the heart and blood vessels to treat hypertension (high blood pressure), angina (chest pain), heart attack, congestive heart failure, arrhythmias, and high cholesterol levels

ACE (ANGIOTENSIN-CONVERTING ENZYME) INHIBITORS

benazepril HCl (Lotensin)
enalaprilat maleate (Vasotec)
fosinopril sodium (Monopril)
lisinopril (Prinivil, Zestril)
quinapril HCl (Accupril)
ramipril (Altace)
valsartan (Diovan)

ANGIOTENSIN II INHIBITORS

irbesartan (Avapro)
losartan potassium (Cozaar, Hyzaar)

BETA BLOCKERS

atenolol (Tenormin)
metoprolol (Lopressor)
nadolol (Corgard)
propranolol HCl

CALCIUM CHANNEL BLOCKERS

amlodipine (Norvasc)
diltiazem (Cardizem)
felodipine (Plendil)
nifedipine (Adalat CC, Procardia)
verapamil HCl

CHOLESTEROL-LOWERING DRUGS

atorvastatin calcium (Lipitor)
cholestyramine resin (Questran)
fluvastatin (Lescol)
lovastatin (Mevacor)
pravastatin sodium (Pravachol)
simvastatin (Zocor)

DIURETICS

furosemide (Lasix)
hydrochlorothiazide
spironolactone (Aldactone)

VASODILATORS

isosorbide mononitrate (Imdur)
nitroglycerin (Nitrostat)

ENDOCRINE DRUGS

Hormones that act in the same manner as naturally occurring hormones and treat disorders of the endocrine glands

ANDROGENS

fluoxymestrone (Halotestin)
methyltestosterone

ANTIANDROGEN

flutamide (Eulexin)

ESTROGENS

conjugated estrogens (Premarin)
estradiol (Climara, Estrace, Estraderm)

ANTIESTROGEN

tamoxifen citrate (Nolvadex)

GLUCOCORTICOIDS

dexamethasone (Decadron)
prednisone (Deltasone)

PROGESTINS

medroxyprogesterone acetate (Cycrin, Provera)
megestrol (Megace)

SERM (SELECTIVE ESTROGEN RECEPTOR MODULATOR)

raloxifene HCl (Evista)

THYROID HORMONES

levothyroxine sodium (Levothroid, Levoxyl, Synthroid)
liothyronine sodium (Cytomel)
liotrix (Thyrolar)

GASTROINTESTINAL DRUGS

Agents for the relief of gastrointestinal disorders and symptoms

ANTACIDS

aluminum and magnesium antacid (Gaviscon)
magnesium antacid (Milk of Magnesia)

ANTIDIARRHEALS

diphenoxylate/atropine (Lomotil)
loperamide (Imodium)
paregoric

ANTINAUSANTS (ANTIEMETICS)

meclizine (Antivert)
metoclopramide (Reglan)
ondansetron (Zofran)
promethazine HCl (Phenergan)
prochlorperazine maleate (Compazine)

ANTIULCER AND ANTI-GERD (GASTROESOPHAGEAL REFLUX DISEASE)

cimetidine (Tagamet)
famotidine (Pepcid)
lansoprazole (Prevacid)
omeprazole (Prilosec)
ranitidine HCl (Zantac)

CATHARTIC

casanthranol and docusate sodium (Peri-Colace)

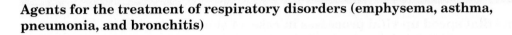

RESPIRATORY DRUGS

Agents for the treatment of respiratory disorders (emphysema, asthma, pneumonia, and bronchitis)

BRONCHODILATORS

albuterol sulfate (Proventil)
epinephrine
ipratropium (Atrovent)
ipratropium bromide and albuterol sulfate (Combivent)
theophylline (Theo-Dur)

STEROIDS

beclomethasone (Vanceril)
flunisolide (AeroBid)
methylprednisolone
triamcinolone (Azmacort)

SEDATIVES/HYPNOTICS

Agents that depress the central nervous system to promote drowsiness and sleep

BARBITURATES

butabarbital (Butisol)
pentobarbital
phenobarbital

BENZODIAZEPINES

lorazepam (Ativan)
temazepam (Restoril)
triazolam (Halcion)

OTHERS

chloral hydrate
zolpidem tartrate (Ambien)

STIMULANTS

Agents that speed up vital processes in case of shock and collapse, increase alertness, and inhibit hyperactive behavior in children

caffeine
dextroamphetamine sulfate (Dexedrine)
methylphenidate (Ritalin)

TRANQUILIZERS

Agents that treat tension, anxiety, and agitation (minor tranquilizers) and psychoses (major tranquilizers)

MINOR

alprazolam (Xanax)
buspirone (BuSpar)
diazepam (Valium)
lorazepam (Ativan)

MAJOR

chlorpromazine (Thorazine)
lithium
olanzapine (Zyprexa)
thioridazine (Mellaril)
trifluoperazine (Stelazine)

DIAGNOSTIC TESTS AND PROCEDURES

RADIOLOGY, ULTRASOUND, AND IMAGING PROCEDURES

In many of the following procedures a *contrast* substance (sometimes referred to as a *dye*) is introduced into or around a body part so that the part can be viewed while x-rays are taken. The contrast substance (often containing barium or iodine) appears dense on the x-ray and outlines the body part that it fills.

The suffix -GRAPHY, meaning "process of recording," is used in many terms describing imaging procedures. The suffix -GRAM, meaning "record," is also used and describes the actual image that is produced by this procedure.

Pronunciation of each term is given with its meaning. The syllable that gets the accent is in **CAPITAL LETTERS.** *Italicized* terms indicate important additional terminology, and terms in SMALL CAPITAL LETTERS are defined elsewhere in this appendix.

ANGIOGRAPHY (an-je-OG-rah-fe) or ANGIOGRAM (AN-je-o-gram): X-ray recording of blood vessels. A contrast substance is injected into blood vessels (veins and arteries), and x-ray pictures are taken of the vessels. In *cerebral angiography,* x-ray pictures are taken of blood vessels in the brain. Angiography is used to detect abnormalities in blood vessels, such as blockage, malformation, and arteriosclerosis. Angiography is performed most frequently to view arteries and is often used interchangeably with *arteriography.*

ARTERIOGRAPHY (ar-ter-e-OG-rah-fe) or ARTERIOGRAM (ar-TER-e-oh-gram): X-ray recording of arteries after injection of a contrast substance into an artery. *Coronary arteriography* is the visualization of arteries that bring blood to the heart muscle.

BARIUM TESTS (BAH-re-um tests): X-ray examinations using a liquid barium mixture to locate disorders in the esophagus *(esophagogram),* duodenum, small intestine *(small bowel follow-through),* and colon *(barium enema).* Taken before or during the examination, barium causes the intestinal tract to stand out in silhouette when viewed through a *fluoroscope* or seen on an x-ray film. The *barium swallow* is used to examine the upper gastrointestinal tract, and the *barium enema* is for examination of the lower gastrointestinal tract.

BARIUM ENEMA: See LOWER GASTROINTESTINAL EXAMINATION and BARIUM TESTS.

BARIUM SWALLOW: See ESOPHAGOGRAPHY and BARIUM TESTS.

CARDIAC CATHETERIZATION (KAR-de-ak cath-eh-ter-i-ZA-shun): Procedure in which a catheter (tube) is passed via vein or artery into the chambers of the heart to measure the blood flow out of the heart and the pressures and oxygen content in the heart chambers. Contrast material is also introduced into heart chambers, and x-ray images are taken to show heart structure.

CEREBRAL ANGIOGRAPHY: See ANGIOGRAPHY.

CHEST X-RAY: An x-ray of the chest that may show infection (as in pneumonia or tuberculosis), emphysema, occupational exposure (asbestosis), lung tumors, or heart enlargement.

CHOLANGIOGRAPHY (kol-an-je-OG-rah-fe) or CHOLANGIOGRAM (kol-AN-je-o-gram): X-ray recording of bile ducts. Contrast material is given by intravenous injection *(I.V. cholangiogram)* and collects in the gallbladder and bile ducts. Also, contrast can be introduced (through the skin) by a percutaneously placed needle inserted into an intrahepatic duct *(percutaneous transhepatic cholangiography).* X-rays are taken of bile ducts to identify obstructions caused by tumors or stones.

COMPUTED TOMOGRAPHY (CT) (kom-PU-ted to-MOG-ra-fe): X-ray images taken to show the body in cross-section. Contrast material may be used (injected into the bloodstream) to highlight structures such as the liver, brain, or blood vessels, and barium can be swallowed to outline gastrointestinal organs. X-ray images, taken as the x-ray tube rotates around the body, are processed by a computer to show "slices" of body tissues, most often within the head, chest, and abdomen.

CORONARY ARTERIOGRAPHY: See ARTERIOGRAPHY.

CYSTOGRAPHY (sis-TOG-rah-fe) or CYSTOGRAM (SIS-to-gram): X-ray recording of the urinary bladder using a contrast medium so that the outline of the urinary bladder can be seen clearly. A contrast substance is injected via catheter into the urethra and urinary bladder, and x-ray images are taken. A *voiding cystourethrogram* is an x-ray image of the urinary tract made while the patient is urinating.

DIGITAL SUBTRACTION ANGIOGRAPHY (DIJ-i-tal sub-TRAK-shun an-je-OG-rah-fe): A unique x-ray technique for viewing blood vessels by taking two images and subtracting one from the other. Images are first taken without contrast and then again after contrast is injected into blood vessels. The first image is then subtracted from the second so that the final image (sharp and precise) shows only contrast-filled blood vessels minus surrounding tissue.

DOPPLER ULTRASOUND (DOP-ler UL-tra-sound): An instrument that focuses sound waves on blood vessels and measured blood flow as echoes bounce off red blood cells. Arteries or veins in the arms, neck, or legs are examined to detect vascular occlusion (blockage) caused by clots or atherosclerosis.

ECHOCARDIOGRAPHY (eh-ko-kar-de-OG-rah-fe) or ECHOCARDIOGRAM (eh-ko-KAR-de-o-gram): Images of the heart produced by introducing high-frequency sound waves through the chest into the heart. The sound waves are reflected back from the heart, and echoes showing heart structure are displayed on a recording machine. It is a highly useful diagnostic tool in the evaluation of diseases of the valves that separate the heart chambers and diseases of the heart muscle.

ECHOENCEPHALOGRAPHY (eh-ko-en-sef-ah-LOG-rah-fe) or ECHOENCEPHALOGRAM (eh-ko-en-SEF-ah-lo-gram): An ultrasound recording of the brain. Sound waves are beamed at the brain, and the echoes that return to the machine are recorded as graphic tracings. Brain tumors and hematomas can be detected by abnormal tracings.

ENDOSCOPIC RETROGRADE CHOLANGIOPANCREATOGRAPHY or ERCP (en-do-SKOP-ik REH-tro-grad kol-an-je-o-pan-kre-ah-TOG-rah-fe): X-ray recording of the bile ducts, pancreas, and pancreatic duct. Radiopaque contrast is injected via a tube through the mouth into the bile and pancreatic ducts, and x-rays are then taken.

ESOPHAGOGRAPHY (eh-sof-ah-GOG-rah-fe) or ESOPHAGOGRAM (eh-SOF-ah-go-gram): X-ray images taken of the esophagus after barium sulfate is swallowed. This test is also called a *barium meal* or BARIUM SWALLOW and is part of an UPPER GASTROINTESTINAL EXAMINATION.

FLUOROSCOPY (flur-OS-ko-pe): An x-ray procedure that uses a fluorescent screen rather than a photographic plate to show images of the body. X-rays that have passed through the body strike a screen covered with a fluorescent substance that emits yellow-green light. Internal organs are seen directly and in motion. Fluoroscopy is used to guide the insertion of catheters and during BARIUM TESTS.

GALLBLADDER ULTRASOUND (GAWL-blah-der UL-tra-sownd): Procedure in which sound waves are used to visualize gallstones. This procedure has replaced cholecystography, which required ingestion of an iodine-based contrast substance.

HYSTEROSALPINGOGRAPHY (his-ter-o-sal-ping-OG-rah-fe) or HYSTEROSALPINGOGRAM (his-ter-o-sal-PING-o-gram): X-ray recording of the uterus and fallopian tubes. Contrast medium is inserted through the vagina into the uterus and fallopian tubes, and x-rays are taken to detect blockage or tumor.

INTRAVENOUS PYELOGRAPHY: See UROGRAPHY.

LOWER GASTROINTESTINAL EXAMINATION (LO-wer gas-tro-in-TES-tin-al ek-zam-ih-NA-shun): X-ray pictures of the colon taken after a liquid contrast substance called barium sulfate is inserted through a plastic tube (enema) into the rectum and large intestine (colon). If tumor is present in the colon, it may appear as an obstruction or irregularity. Also known as a BARIUM ENEMA.

LYMPHANGIOGRAPHY (limfan-je-OG-rah-fe) or LYMPHANGIOGRAM (LIMFAN-je-o-gram): X-ray recording of the lymph nodes and lymph vessels after contrast is injected into lymphatic vessels in the feet. The contrast medium travels upward through the lymphatic vessels of the pelvis, abdomen, and chest and outlines the architecture of lymph nodes in all areas of the body. This procedure is used to detect tumors within the lymphatic system. It is also known as *lymphography*.

LYMPHOGRAPHY: See LYMPHANGIOGRAPHY.

MAGNETIC RESONANCE IMAGING (mag-NET-ik REZ-o-nans IM-a-jing) or MRI: Magnetic waves and radiofrequency pulses, not x-rays, used to create an image of body organs. The images can be taken in several planes of the body—frontal, sagittal (side), and transverse (cross-section)—and are particularly useful for studying tumors of the brain and spinal cord. Magnetic waves beamed at the heart give information about congenital heart disease and cardiac lesions before surgery.

MAMMOGRAPHY (MAMOG-rah-fe) or MAMMOGRAM (MAM-o-gram): X-ray recording of the breast. X-rays of low voltage are beamed at the breast, and images are produced. Mammography is used to detect abnormalities in breast tissue, such as early breast cancer.

MYELOGRAPHY (mi-eh-LOG-rah-fe) or MYELOGRAM (MI-eh-lo-gram): X-ray recording of the spinal cord. X-rays are taken of the fluid-filled space surrounding the spinal cord after a contrast medium is injected into the subarachnoid space (between the membranes surrounding the spinal cord) at the lumbar level of the back. Myelography detects tumors or ruptured, "slipped," discs that lie between the backbones (vertebrae) and press on the spinal cord.

PYELOGRAPHY or PYELOGRAM: See UROGRAPHY.

SMALL BOWEL FOLLOW-THROUGH: See BARIUM TESTS and UPPER GASTROINTESTINAL EXAMINATION.

TOMOGRAPHY (to-MOG-rah-fe) or TOMOGRAM (TO-mo-gram): X-ray recording that shows an organ in depth. Several pictures ("slices") are taken of an organ by moving the x-ray tube and film in sequence to blur out certain regions and bring others into sharper focus. Tomograms of the kidney and lung are examples.

ULTRASONOGRAPHY (ul-trah-so-NOG-rah-fe) or ULTRASONOGRAM (ul-trah-SON-o-gram): Images produced by beaming sound waves into the body and capturing the echoes that bounce off organs. These echoes are then processed to produce an image showing the difference between fluid and solid masses and the general position of organs.

UPPER GASTROINTESTINAL EXAMINATION (UP-er gas-tro-in-TES-tin-al ek-zam-ih-NA-shun): X-ray pictures taken of the esophagus *(barium meal* or BARIUM SWALLOW), duodenum, and small intestine after a liquid contrast substance called barium sulfate is swallowed. In a SMALL BOWEL FOLLOW-THROUGH, pictures are taken at increasing time intervals to follow the progress of barium through the small intestine. Identification of obstructions or ulcers is possible.

UROGRAPHY (u-ROG-rah-fe) or UROGRAM (UR-o-gram): X-ray recording of the kidney and urinary tract. If x-rays are taken after contrast medium is injected intravenously, the procedure is called *intravenous urography (descending* or *excretion urography)* or *intravenous pyelography (IVP).* If x-rays are taken after injection of contrast medium into the bladder through the urethra, the procedure is *retrograde urography* or *retrograde pyelography.* PYEL/O- means "renal pelvis" (the collecting chamber of the kidney).

NUCLEAR MEDICINE SCANS

In the following diagnostic tests, radioactive material *(radioisotope)* is injected, inhaled, or swallowed and then detected by a scanning device in the organ in which it accumulates. X-rays, ultrasound, or magnetic waves are not used.

The pronunciation of each term is given with its meaning. The syllable that gets the accent is in **CAPITAL LETTERS.**

BONE SCAN: Procedure in which a radioactive substance is injected intravenously and its uptake in bones is detected by a scanning device. Tumors in bone can be detected by increased uptake of the radioactive material in the areas of the lesions.

BRAIN SCAN: Procedure in which a radioactive substance is injected intravenously. It collects in any lesion that disturbs the natural barrier that exists between blood vessels and normal brain tissue (blood-brain barrier), allowing the radioactive substance to enter the brain tissue. A scanning device detects the presence of the radioactive substance and thus can identify an area of tumor, abscess, or hematoma.

GALLIUM SCAN (GAL-le-um skan):   Procedure in which radioactive gallium (gallium citrate) is injected into the bloodstream and is detected in the body using a scanning device that produces an image of the areas where gallium collects. The gallium collects in areas of certain tumors (Hodgkin disease, hematoma, various adenocarcinomas) and in areas of infection.

MUGA SCAN (MUH-gah skan):   Test that uses radioactive technetium to detect a heart attack (myocardial infarction). Also called *technetium-99m ventriculography* or *multiple-gated acquisition* scan.

POSITRON EMISSION TOMOGRAPHY (POS-i-tron e-MISH-un to-MOG-rah-fe) or PET scan: Procedure in which radioactive substances (oxygen and glucose are used) that release radioactive particles called positrons are injected into the body and travel to specialized areas such as the brain and heart. Because of the way that the positrons are released, cross-sectional color pictures can be made showing the location of the radioactive substance. This test is used to study disorders of the brain and to diagnose strokes, epilepsy, schizophrenia, coronary artery disease, and migraine headaches.

PULMONARY PERFUSION SCAN (PUL-mo-ner-e per-FU-shun skan): Procedure in which radioactive particles are injected intravenously and travel rapidly to areas of the lung that are adequately filled with blood. Regions of obstructed blood flow caused by tumor, blood clot, swelling, and inflammation can be seen as nonradioactive areas on the scan.

PULMONARY VENTILATION SCAN (PUL-mo-ner-e ven-ti-LA-shun skan): Procedure in which radioactive gas is inhaled and a special camera detects its presence in the lungs. The scan is used to detect lung segments that fail to fill with the radioactive gas. Lack of filling is usually due to diseases that obstruct the bronchial tubes and air sacs. This scan is also used in the evaluation of lung function before surgery.

THALLIUM-201 SCINTIGRAPHY (THAL-e-um-201 SIN-tih-gra-fe): Procedure in which thallium-201 in injected into a vein and images of blood flow through heart muscle are recorded as a person performs an exercise test. *Sestamibi scans (ETT-MIBI)* are also used to assess the status of blood flow through heart muscle during an exercise stress test.

THYROID SCAN (THI-royd skan): Procedure in which a radioactive iodine chemical is injected intravenously and collects in the thyroid gland. A scanning device detects the radioactive substance in the gland, measuring it and producing an image of the gland. The increased or decreased activity of the gland is demonstrated by the gland's capacity to use the radioactive iodine. A thyroid scan is used to evaluate the position, size, and functioning of the thyroid gland.

CLINICAL PROCEDURES

The following procedures are performed on patients to establish a correct diagnosis of an abnormal condition. In some instances, the procedure may also be used to treat the condition.

Pronunciation of each term is given with its meaning. The syllable that gets the accent is in **CAPITAL LETTERS.** Terms in SMALL CAPITAL LETTERS are defined elsewhere in the appendix. *Italicized* terms are additional important terminology.

ABDOMINOCENTESIS (ab-dom-in-o-sen-TE-sis): See PARACENTESIS.

AMNIOCENTESIS (am-ne-o-sen-TE-sis): Surgical puncture to remove fluid from the sac (amnion) that surrounds the fetus in the uterus. The fluid contains cells from the fetus that can be examined under a microscope for chromosomal analysis.

ASPIRATION (as-peh-RA-shun): The withdrawal of fluid by suction through a needle or tube. The term "aspiration pneumonia" refers to an infection caused by inhalation into the lungs of food or an object.

AUDIOMETRY (aw-de-OM-eh-tre): A test using sound waves of various frequencies (e.g., 500 Hz) up to 8000 Hz, which quantifies the extent and type of hearing loss. An *audiogram* is the record produced by this test.

AUSCULTATION (aw-skul-TA-shun): The process of listening for sounds produced within the body. This is most often performed with the aid of a stethoscope to determine the condition of the chest or abdominal organs or to detect the fetal heart beat.

BIOPSY (BI-op-se):   The removal of a piece of tissue from the body and subsequent examination of the tissue under a microscope. The procedure is performed by means of a surgical knife, by needle aspiration, or via endoscopic removal (using a special forceps-like instrument inserted through a hollow flexible tube.) An *excisional biopsy* means that the entire tissue to be examined is removed. An *incisional biopsy* is the removal of only a small amount of tissue, and a *needle biopsy* indicates that tissue is pierced with a hollow needle and fluid is withdrawn for microscopic examination.

BONE MARROW BIOPSY (bon MAH-ro BI-op-se):   The removal of a small amount of bone marrow. The cells are then examined under a microscope. Often the hip bone (iliac crest) is used, and the biopsy is helpful in determining the number and type of blood cells in the bone marrow. Also called a bone marrow ASPIRATION.

BRONCHOSCOPY (brong-KOS-ko-pe):   The insertion of a flexible tube (endoscope) into the airway. The lining of the bronchial tubes can be seen, and tissue may be removed for biopsy. The tube is usually inserted through the mouth but can also be directly inserted into the airway during MEDIASTINOSCOPY. Sedation is required for this procedure.

CHORIONIC VILLUS SAMPLING (kor-e-ON-ik VIL-us SAM-pling):   Removal and microscopic analysis of a small piece of placental tissue to detect fetal abnormalities.

COLONOSCOPY (ko-lon-OS-ko-pe):   The insertion of a flexible tube (endoscope) through the rectum into the colon for visual examination. Biopsy samples may be taken and benign growths, such as polyps, can be removed through the endoscope. The removal of a polyp is called a polypectomy (pol-eh-PEK-to-me).

COLPOSCOPY (kol-POS-ko-pe):   The inspection of the cervix through the insertion of a special microscope into the vagina. The vaginal walls are held apart by a speculum so that the cervix (entrance to the uterus) can come into view.

CONIZATION (ko-nih-ZA-shun):   The removal of a cone-shaped sample of uterine cervix tissue. This sample is then examined under a microscope for evidence of cancerous growth. The special shape of the tissue sample allows the pathologist to examine the transitional zone of the cervix, where cancers are most likely to develop.

CULDOCENTESIS (kul-do-sen-TE-sis):   The insertion of a thin, hollow needle through the vagina into the cul-de-sac, the space between the rectum and the uterus. Fluid is withdrawn and analyzed for evidence of cancerous cells, infection, or blood cells.

CYSTOSCOPY (sis-TOS-ko-pe):   The insertion of a thin tube or cystoscope (endoscope) into the urethra and then into the urinary bladder to visualize the bladder. A biopsy of the urinary bladder can be performed through the cystoscope.

DIGITAL RECTAL EXAMINATION (DIG-ih-tal REK-tal eks-am-ih-NA-shun): Procedure in which the physician inserts a gloved finger into the rectum. This procedure is used to detect rectal cancer and as a primary method of detection of prostate cancer. The abbreviation is *DRG*.

DILATION AND CURETTAGE (di-LA-shun and kur-eh-TAJ): Procedure in which a series of probes of increasing size is systematically inserted through the vagina into the opening of the cervix. The cervix is thus dilated (widened) so that a curette (spoon-shaped instrument) can be inserted to remove tissue from the lining of the uterus. The tissue is then examined under a microscope. The abbreviation for this procedure is *D&C*.

ELECTROCARDIOGRAPHY (e-lek-tro-kar-de-OG-rah-fe): The connection of electrodes (wires or "leads") to the body to record electric impulses from the heart. The *electrocardiogram* is the actual record produced, and it is useful in discovering abnormalities in heart rhythms and diagnosing heart disorders. The abbreviation is *EKG* or *ECG*.

ELECTROENCEPHALOGRAPHY (e-lek-tro-en-sef-ah-LOG-rah-fe): The connection of electrodes (wires or "leads") to the scalp to record electricity coming from within the brain. The *electroencephalogram* is the actual record produced. It is useful in the diagnosis and monitoring of epilepsy and other brain lesions and in the investigation of neurological disorders. It is also used to evaluate patients in coma (brain inactivity) and in the study of sleep disorders. The abbreviation is *EEG*.

ELECTROMYOGRAPHY (e-lek-tro-mi-OG-rah-fe): The insertion of needle electrodes into muscle to record electrical activity. This procedure detects injuries and diseases that affect muscles and nerves. The abbreviation is *EMG*.

ENDOSCOPY (en-DOS-ko-pe): The insertion of a thin, tube-like instrument (endoscope) into an organ or cavity. The endoscope is placed through a natural opening (the mouth or anus) or into a surgical incision, such as through the abdominal wall. Endoscopes contain bundles of glass fibers that carry light (fiberoptic); some instruments are equipped with a small forceps-like device that withdraws a sample of tissue for microscopic study (biopsy). Examples of endoscopy are BRONCHOSCOPY, COLONOSCOPY, ESOPHAGOSCOPY, GASTROSCOPY, and LAPAROSCOPY.

ESOPHAGOGASTRODUODENOSCOPY (eh-SOF-ah-go-GAS-tro-du-o-den-NOS-ko-pe): The insertion of an endoscope through the mouth into the esophagus, stomach, and first part of the small intestine. Also called *EGD*.

ESOPHAGOSCOPY (eh-sof-ah-GOS-ko-pe): The insertion of an endoscope through the mouth and throat into the esophagus. Visual examination of the esophagus to detect ulcers, tumors, or other lesions is thus possible.

EXCISIONAL BIOPSY (ek-SIZ-in-al BI-op-se): See BIOPSY.

FROZEN SECTION (fro-zen SEK-shun): The quick preparation of a biopsy sample for examination during an actual surgical procedure. Tissue is taken from the operating room to the pathology laboratory and frozen. It is then thinly sliced and immediately examined under a microscope to determine if the sample is benign or malignant and to determine the status of margins.

GASTROSCOPY (gas-TROS-ko-pe): The insertion of an endoscope through the esophagus into the stomach for visual examination and/or biopsy of the stomach. When the upper portion of the small intestine is also visualized, the procedure is called *EGD* or ESOPHAGOGASTRODUODENOSCOPY.

HOLTER MONITOR (HOL-ter ECG MON-ih-ter): The electrocardiographic record of heart activity over an extended period of time. The Holter monitor is worn by the patient as he/she performs normal daily activities. It detects and aids in the management of heart rhythm abnormalities. Also called *ambulatory electrocardiograph.*

HYSTEROSCOPY (his-ter-OS-ko-pe): The insertion of an endoscope into the uterus for visual examination.

INCISIONAL BIOPSY (in-SIZ-in-al BI-op-se): See BIOPSY.

LAPAROSCOPY (lap-ah-ROS-ko-pe): The insertion of an endoscope into the abdomen. After the patient receives a local anesthetic, a laparoscope is inserted through an incision in the abdominal wall. This procedure gives the doctor a view of the abdominal cavity, the surface of the liver and spleen, and the pelvic region. Laparoscopy is used to perform fallopian tube ligation as a means of preventing pregnancy.

LARYNGOSCOPY (lah-rin-GOS-ko-pe): The insertion of an endoscope into the airway to visually examine the voice box (larynx). A laryngoscope transmits a magnified image of the larynx through a system of lenses and mirrors. The procedure can reveal tumors and explain changes in the voice. Sputum samples and tissue biopsies are obtained by using brushes or forceps attached to the laryngoscope.

MEDIASTINOSCOPY (me-de-ah-sti-NOS-ko-pe): The insertion of an endoscope into the mediastinum (space in the chest between the lungs and in front of the heart). A mediastinoscope is inserted through a small incision in the neck while the patient is under anesthesia. This procedure is used to biopsy lymph nodes and to examine other structures within the mediastinum.

NEEDLE BIOPSY (NE-dl BI-op-se): See BIOPSY.

OPHTHALMOSCOPIC EXAM (of-thal-mo-SKOP-ic ek-ZAM): A physician uses an *ophthalmoscope* to look directly into the eye, evaluating the optic nerve, retina, and blood vessels in the back of the eye and the lens in the front of the eye for cataracts. Also called *ophthalmoscopy.*

OTOSCOPIC EXAM (o-to-SKOP-ic ek-ZAM): A physician uses an *otoscope* inserted into the ear canal to check for obstructions (e.g., wax), infection, fluid, and eardrum perforations or scarring. Also called *otoscopy.*

PALPATION (pal-PA-shun): Examination by touch. This is a technique of manual physical examination by which a doctor feels underlying tissues and organs through the skin.

PAP SMEAR (pap smer):   The insertion of a cotton swab or wooden spatula into the vagina to obtain a sample of cells from the outer surface of the cervix (neck of the uterus). The cells are then smeared on a glass slide, preserved, and sent to the laboratory for microscopic examination. This test for cervical cancer was developed and named after the late Dr. George Papanicolaou. Results are reported as a Grade I to IV (I = normal, II = inflammatory, III = suspicious of malignancy, IV = malignancy).

PARACENTESIS (pah-rah-sen-TE-sis):   Surgical puncture of the membrane surrounding the abdomen (peritoneum) to remove fluid from the abdominal cavity. Fluid is drained for analysis and to prevent its accumulation in the abdomen. Also known as ABDOMINOCENTESIS.

PELVIC EXAM (PEL-vik ek-ZAM):   Physician examines female sex organs and checks the uterus and ovaries for enlargement, cysts, tumors, or abnormal bleeding. This is also known as an "internal exam."

PERCUSSION (per-KUSH-un):   The technique of striking a part of the body with short, sharp taps of the fingers to determine the size, density, and position of the underlying parts by the sound obtained. Percussion is commonly used on the abdomen to examine the liver.

PROCTOSIGMOIDOSCOPY (prok-to-sig-moy-DOS-ko-pe):   The insertion of an endoscope through the anus to examine the first 10 to 12 inches of the rectum and colon. When the sigmoid colon is visualized using a longer endoscope, the procedure is called *sigmoidoscopy*. The procedure detects polyps, malignant tumors, and sources of bleeding.

PULMONARY FUNCTION TEST (PUL-mo-ner-e FUNG-shun test):   The measurement of the air taken into and exhaled from the lungs by means of an instrument called a *spirometer*. The test may be abnormal in patients with asthma, chronic bronchitis, emphysema, and occupational exposures to asbestos, chemicals, and dusts.

SIGMOIDOSCOPY (sig-moy-DOS-ko-pe):   See PROCTOSIGMOIDOSCOPY.

STRESS TEST (stres test): An electrocardiogram taken during exercise. It may reveal hidden heart disease or confirm the cause of cardiac symptoms.

THORACENTESIS (thor-ah-sen-TE-sis):   The insertion of a needle into the chest to remove fluid from the space surrounding the lungs (pleural cavity). After injection of a local anesthetic, a hollow needle is placed through the skin and muscles of the back and into the space between the lungs and chest wall. Fluid is then withdrawn by applying suction. Excess fluid *(pleural effusion)* may be a sign of infection or malignancy. This procedure is used to diagnose conditions, to drain a pleural effusion, or to re-expand a collapsed lung *(atelectasis)*.

THORACOSCOPY (tho-rah-KOS-ko-pe):   The insertion of an endoscope through an incision in the chest to visually examine the surface of the lungs.

LABORATORY TESTS

The following laboratory tests are performed on samples of a patient's blood, *plasma* (fluid portion of the blood), *serum* (plasma minus clotting proteins and produced after blood has clotted), urine, feces, *sputum* (mucus coughed up from the lungs), *cerebrospinal fluid* (fluid within the spaces around the spinal cord and brain), and skin.

Pronunciation of each term is given with its meaning. The syllable that gets the accent is in **CAPITAL LETTERS.** Terms in SMALL CAPITAL LETTERS are defined elsewhere in the appendix. *Italicized* terms are additional important terminology.

ACID PHOSPHATASE (AH-sid FOS-fah-tas):   Measurement of the amount of an enzyme called *acid phosphatase* in serum. Enzyme levels are elevated in metastatic prostate cancer. Moderate elevations of this enzyme occur in diseases of bone and when breast cancer cells invade bone tissue.

ALBUMIN (al-BU-min):   Measurement of the amount of albumin (protein) in both the serum and the urine. A decrease of albumin in serum indicates disease of the kidneys, malnutrition, or liver disease or may occur in extensive loss of protein in the gut or from the skin, as in a burn. The presence of albumin in the urine *(albuminuria)* indicates malfunction of the kidney.

ALKALINE PHOSPHATASE (AL-kah-lin FOS-fah-tas):   Measurement of the amount of *alkaline phosphatase* (an enzyme found on cell membranes) in serum. Levels are elevated in liver diseases (such as hepatitis and hepatoma) and in bone disease and bone cancer. The laboratory symbol is *alk phos.*

ALPHA-FETOPROTEIN (al-fa-fe-to-PRO-teen):   Determination of the presence of a protein called alpha-globulin in serum. The protein is normally present in the serum of the fetus, infant, and pregnant woman. In fetuses with abnormalities of the brain and spinal cord, the protein leaks into the amniotic fluid surrounding the fetus and is an indicator of spinal tube defect (spina bifida) or anencephaly (lack of brain development). High levels are found in patients with cancer of the liver and other malignancies (testicular and ovarian cancers). Serum levels monitor the effectiveness of cancer treatment. Elevated levels are also seen in benign liver disease such as cirrhosis and viral hepatitis. The laboratory symbol is *AFP.*

ALT: Measurement of the amount of the enzyme called *alanine transaminase* in serum. The enzyme is normally present in blood but accumulates in high amounts with damage to liver cells. Also called *SGPT.*

ANA: See ANTINUCLEAR ANTIBODY TEST.

ANTINUCLEAR ANTIBODY TEST (an-tih-NU-kle-ar AN-tih-bod-e test): Procedure in which a sample of plasma is tested for the presence of antibodies that are found in patients with systemic lupus erythematosus. Laboratory symbol is *ANA.*

AST: Measurement of the enzyme *aspartate transaminase* in serum. The enzyme is normally present in blood but accumulates when there is damage to the heart or to liver cells. Also called *SGOT.*

BENCE JONES PROTEIN (BENS jonz PRO-ten):   Measurement of the presence of the Bence Jones protein in serum or urine. Bence Jones protein is a fragment of a normal serum protein, an immunoglobulin, produced by cancerous bone marrow cells (myeloma cells). Normally it is not found in either blood or urine, but in *multiple myeloma* (a malignant condition of bone marrow) high levels of Bence Jones protein are detected in urine and serum.

BILIRUBIN (bil-ih-RU-bin):   Measurement of the amount of bilirubin, an orange-brown pigment, in serum and urine. Bilirubin is derived from hemoglobin, the oxygen-carrying protein in red blood cells. Its presence in high concentration in serum and urine causes *jaundice* (yellow coloration of the skin) and may indicate disease of the liver, obstruction of bile ducts, or a type of anemia that leads to excessive destruction of red blood cells.

BLOOD CHEMISTRY PROFILE: A comprehensive blood test that is a biochemical examination of various substances in the blood using a computerized laboratory analyzer. Tests include calcium (bones), phosphorus (bones), urea (kidney), creatinine (kidney), bilirubin (liver), AST or SGOT (liver and heart muscle) and ALT or SGPT (liver), alkaline phosphatase (liver and bone), globulin (liver and immune disorders), and albumin (liver and kidney). Also called SMA or sequential multiple analysis. SMA-6, SMA-12, and SMA-18 indicate the number of blood elements tested.

BLOOD CULTURE (blud KUL-chur):   Test to determine whether infection is present in the bloodstream. A sample of blood is added to a special medium (food) that promotes the growth of microorganisms. The medium is then examined by a medical technologist for evidence of bacteria or other microbes.

BLOOD UREA NITROGEN (blud u-RE-ah NI-tro-jen):   Measurement of the amount of urea (nitrogen-containing waste material) in serum. A high level of serum urea indicates poor kidney function, since it is the kidney's job to remove urea from the bloodstream and filter it into urine. The laboratory symbol is *BUN*.

CALCIUM (KAL-se-um):   Measurement of the amount of calcium in serum, plasma, or whole blood. Low blood levels are associated with abnormal functioning of nerves and muscles, and high blood levels indicate loss of calcium from bones, excessive intake of calcium, disease of the parathyroid glands, or cancer. The laboratory symbol is *Ca*.

CARBON DIOXIDE (KAR-bon di-OK-side):   Blood test to measure the gas produced in tissues and eliminated by the lungs. Abnormal levels may reflect lung disorders. The laboratory symbol is CO_2.

CARCINOEMBRYONIC ANTIGEN (kar-sih-no-em-bree-ON-ik AN-ti-jen):   A plasma test for a protein normally found in the blood of human fetuses and produced in healthy adults only in a very small amount, if at all. High levels of this antigen may be a sign of one of a variety of cancers, especially colon or pancreatic cancer. This test is used to monitor the response of patients to cancer treatment. The laboratory abbreviation is *CEA*.

CEREBROSPINAL FLUID (seh-re-bro-SPI-nal FLU-id):   Measurement of cerebrospinal fluid for protein, sugar, and blood cells. The fluid is also cultured to detect microorganisms. Chemical tests are performed on specimens of the fluid removed by *lumbar puncture*. Abnormal conditions such as meningitis, brain tumor, and encephalitis are detected. The laboratory abbreviation is *CSF.*

CHOLESTEROL (ko-LES-ter-ol):   Measurement of the amount of cholesterol (substance found in animal fats and oils, egg yolks, and milk) in serum or plasma. Normal values vary for age and diet; levels above 200 mg/dl indicate a need for further testing and efforts to reduce cholesterol level, since high levels are associated with hardening of arteries and heart disease. Blood is also tested for the presence of a lipoprotein substance that is a combination of cholesterol and protein. High levels of (optimum level is 60 to 100 mg/dL) *HDL* (high-density lipoprotein) cholesterol in the blood are beneficial, since HDL cholesterol promotes the removal and excretion of excess cholesterol from the body, whereas high levels of low-density lipoprotein *(LDL)* are associated with the development of atherosclerosis (optimum level is 100 mg/dl or less).

COMPLETE BLOOD COUNT: Determinations of the numbers of leukocytes (white blood cells), erythrocytes (red blood cells), and platelets (clotting cells). The CBC is useful in diagnosing anemia, infection, and blood cell disorders, such as leukemia.

CREATINE KINASE (KRE-ah-tin KI-nas):   Measurement of levels of creatine kinase, a blood enzyme. Creatine kinase is normally found in heart muscle, brain tissue, and skeletal muscle. The presence of one form *(isoenzyme)* of creatine kinase (either CK-MB or CK2) in the blood is strongly indicative of recent myocardial infarction (heart attack), since the enzyme is released from heart muscle when the muscle is damaged or dying.

CREATININE (kre-AT-tih-nin):   Measurement of the amount of creatinine, a nitrogen-containing waste material, in serum or plasma. It is the most reliable test for kidney function. Since creatinine is normally produced as a protein breakdown product in muscle and is excreted by the kidney in urine, an elevation in the creatinine level in the blood indicates a disturbance of kidney function. Elevations are also seen in high-protein diets and dehydration.

CREATININE CLEARANCE (kre-AT-tih-nin KLER-ans):   Measurement of the rate at which creatinine is cleared (filtered) by the kidneys from the blood. A low creatinine clearance indicates that the kidneys are not functioning effectively to clear creatinine from the bloodstream and filter it into urine.

CULTURE (KUL-chur):   Identification of microorganisms in a special laboratory medium (fluid, solid, or semisolid material). In *sensitivity* tests, culture plates containing a specific microorganism are prepared, and antibiotic-containing disks are applied to the culture surface. After overnight incubation, the area surrounding the disk (where growth was inhibited) is measured to determine whether the antibiotic is effective against the specific organism.

DIFFERENTIAL (di-fer-EN-shul):   See WHITE BLOOD CELL COUNT.

ELECTROLYTES (e-LEK-tro-litz):   Determination of the concentration of *electrolytes* (chemical substances capable of conducting an electric current) in serum or whole blood. When dissolved in water, electrolytes break apart into charged particles *(ions)*. The positively charged electrolytes are *sodium* (Na^+), *potassium* (K^+), *calcium* (Ca^{++}), and *magnesium* (Mg^{++}). The negatively charged electrolytes are *chloride* (Cl^-) and *bicarbonate* (HCO^{3-}). These charged particles should be present at all times for proper functioning of cells. An electrolyte imbalance occurs when serum concentration is either too high or too low. Calcium balance can affect the bones, kidneys, gastrointestinal tract, and neuromuscular activity, and sodium balance affects blood pressure, nerve functioning, and fluid levels surrounding cells. Potassium balance affects heart and muscular activity.

ELECTROPHORESIS: See SERUM PROTEIN ELECTROPHORESIS.

ELISA (eh-LI-zah):   A laboratory assay (test) for the presence of antibodies to the AIDS virus. If a patient tests positive, it is likely that his/her blood contains the AIDS virus (HIV or human immunodeficiency virus). The presence of the virus stimulates white blood cells to make antibodies that are detected by the ELISA assay. This is the first test done to detect AIDS infection and is followed by a WESTERN BLOT test to confirm the results. ELISA is an acronym for *enzyme-l*inked *i*mmuno*s*orbent *a*ssay.

ERYTHROCYTE SEDIMENTATION RATE (eh-RITH-ro-sit sed-ih-men-TA-shun rat):   Measurement of the rate at which red blood cells (erythrocytes) in well-mixed venous blood settle to the bottom (sediment) of a test tube. If the rate of sedimentation is markedly slow (elevated sed rate), it may indicate inflammatory conditions, such as rheumatoid arthritis, or conditions that produce excessive proteins in the blood. Laboratory symbols are *ESR* and *sed rate*.

ESTRADIOL (es-tra-DI-ol):   A test for the concentration of estradiol, which is a form of estrogen (female hormone) in serum, plasma, or urine.

ESTROGEN RECEPTOR ASSAY (ES-tro-jen re-SEP-tor AS-a):   Test, performed at the time of a biopsy, to determine whether a sample of tumor contains an estrogen receptor protein. The protein, if present on breast cancer cells, combines with estrogen, allowing estrogen to promote the growth of the tumor. Thus, if an estrogen receptor assay test is positive (the protein is present), then treatment with an anti-estrogen drug would retard tumor growth. If the assay is negative (the protein is not present), then the tumor would not be affected by anti-estrogen drug treatment.

GLOBULIN (GLOB-u-lin):   Measurement (in serum) of proteins that bind to and destroy foreign substances (antigens). Globulins are made by cells of the immune system. *Gamma globulin* is one type of globulin that contains antibodies to fight disease.

GLUCOSE (GLU-kos):   Measurement of the amount of glucose (sugar) in serum and plasma. High levels of glucose *(hyperglycemia)* indicate diseases such as diabetes mellitus and hyperthyroidism. Glucose is also measured in urine, and its presence indicates diabetes mellitus.

GLUCOSE TOLERANCE TEST (GLU-kos TOL-er-ans test):   Test to determine how the body uses glucose. In the first part of this test, blood and urine samples are taken after the patient has fasted. Then a solution of glucose is given by mouth. A half hour after the glucose is taken, blood and urine samples are obtained again, and are collected every hour for 4 to 5 hours. This test can indicate abnormal conditions such as diabetes mellitus, hypoglycemia, and liver or adrenal gland dysfunction.

HEMATOCRIT (he-MAT-o-krit):   Measurement of the percentage of red blood cells in the blood. The normal range is 40% to 50% in males and 37% to 47% in females. A low hematocrit indicates anemia. The laboratory symbol is *Hct*.

HEMOCCULT TEST (he-mo-o-KULT test):   Examination of small sample of stool for otherwise inapparent occult (hidden) traces of blood. The sample is placed on the surface of a collection kit and reacts with a chemical (e.g., guaiac). A positive result may indicate bleeding from polyps, ulcers, or malignant tumors. This is an important screening test for colon cancer. Also called a STOOL GUAIAC TEST.

HEMOGLOBIN ASSAY (HE-mo-glo-bin AS-a):   Measurement of the concentration of hemoglobin in blood. The normal blood hemoglobin ranges are 13.5 to 18.0 gm/dl in adult males and 12.0 to 16.0 gm/dl in adult females. The laboratory symbol is *Hgb*.

HUMAN CHORIONIC GONADOTROPIN (HU-man kor-e-ON-ik go-nad-o-TRO-pin):   Measurement of the concentration of human chorionic gonadotropin (a hormone secreted by cells of the fetal placenta) in urine. It is detected in urine within days after fertilization of egg and sperm cells and provides the basis of the most commonly used pregnancy test. The laboratory symbol is *hCG*.

IMMUNOASSAY (im-u-no-AS-a):   A method of testing blood and urine for the concentration of various chemicals, such as hormones, drugs, or proteins. The technique makes use of the immunological reaction between antigens and antibodies. An *assay* is a determination of the amount of any particular substance in a mixture.

LIPID TESTS (LIP-id tests):   Lipids are fatty substances such as cholesterol and triglycerides. See CHOLESTEROL and TRIGLYCERIDES.

LIPOPROTEIN TESTS (li-po-PRO-teen tests):   See CHOLESTEROL.

LIVER FUNCTION TESTS (LIV-er FUNG-shun tests):   See ALKALINE PHOSPHATASE, BILIRUBIN, ALT, and AST.

OCCULT BLOOD TEST: See HEMOCCULT TEST.

PKU TEST: Test that determines whether the urine of a newborn baby contains substances called *phenylketones*. If so, the condition is called *phenylketonuria (PKU)*. Phenylketonuria occurs in infants born lacking a specific enzyme. If the enzyme is missing, high levels of *phenylalanine* (an amino acid) accumulate in the blood, affecting the infant's brain and causing mental retardation. This situation is prevented by placing the infant on a special diet that prevents accumulation of phenylalanine in the bloodstream.

PLATELET COUNT (PLAT-let kownt):   Determination of the number of clotting cells (platelets) in a sample of blood.

POTASSIUM (po-TAHS-e-um):   Measurement of the concentration of potassium in serum. Potassium combines with other minerals (such as calcium) and is an important chemical for proper functioning of muscles, especially the heart muscle. The laboratory symbol is K^+. See also ELECTROLYTES.

PROGESTERONE RECEPTOR ASSAY (pro-JES-teh-rone re-SEP-tor AS-a):   Test to determines whether a sample of tumor contains a progesterone receptor protein. A positive test identifies when tumor would be responsive to anti-progesterone hormone therapy.

PROSTATE-SPECIFIC ANTIGEN (PROS-tat spe-SI-fic AN-ti-jen):   Blood test that measures the amount of an antigen elevated in all patients with prostatic cancer and in some with an inflamed prostate gland. The laboratory symbol is *PSA*.

PROTEIN ELECTROPHORESIS: See SERUM PROTEIN ELECTROPHORESIS.

PROTHROMBIN TIME (pro-THROM-bin tim):   Measurement of the activity of factors in the blood that participate in clotting. Deficiency of any of these factors can lead to a prolonged prothrombin time and difficulty in blood clotting. The test is important as a monitor for patients taking anticoagulants, substances that block the activity of blood clotting factors and increase the risk of bleeding.

PSA: See PROSTATE-SPECIFIC ANTIGEN.

RED BLOOD CELL COUNT: Test in which the number of erythrocytes in a sample of blood is counted. A low red blood cell count may indicate anemia. A high count can indicate *polycythemia vera.*

RHEUMATOID FACTOR (ROO-mah-toyd FAK-tor):   Detection of the abnormal protein *rheumatoid factor* in the serum. It is found in patients with rheumatoid arthritis.

SERUM PROTEIN ELECTROPHORESIS (SE-rum PRO-teen e-lek-tro-for-E-sis):   A procedure that separates proteins using an electric current. The material tested, such as serum, containing various proteins, is placed on paper or gel or in liquid, and under the influence of an electric current, the proteins separate (-PHORESIS means "separation") so that they can be identified and measured. The procedure is also known as *protein electrophoresis.*

SGOT: See AST.

SGPT: See ALT.

SKIN TESTS: Tests in which substances are applied to the skin or injected under the skin and the reaction of immune cells in the skin is observed. These tests detect a person's sensitivity to substances such as dust or pollen. They can also indicate if a person has been exposed to the bacteria that cause tuberculosis or diphtheria.

SODIUM: See ELECTROLYTES.

SMA: See BLOOD CHEMISTRY PROFILE.

SPUTUM TEST (SPU-tum test):   Examination of mucus coughed up from a patient's lungs. The sputum is examined microscopically and chemically and is cultured for the presence of microorganisms.

STOOL GUAIAC TEST (stool GWI-ak test): See HEMOCCULT TEST.

THYROID FUNCTION TESTS (THI-royd FUNG-shun tests): Tests that measure the levels of thyroid hormones, such as *thyroxine* (T_4) and *triiodothyronine* (T_3), in serum. *Thyroid-stimulating hormone (TSH),* which is produced by the pituitary gland and stimulates the release of T_4 and T_3 from the thyroid gland, can also be measured in serum. These tests aid in the diagnosis of hypothyroidism and hyperthyroidism and are helpful in monitoring response to thyroid treatment.

TRIGLYCERIDE (tri-GLIS-er-ide): Determination of the amount of *triglycerides* (fats) in the serum. Elevated triglyceride levels are considered an important risk factor for the development of heart disease.

URIC ACID (UR-ik AS-id): Measurement of the amount of uric acid (a nitrogen-containing waste material) in the serum and urine. High serum levels indicate a type of arthritis called *gout.* In gout, uric acid accumulates as crystals in joints and in tissues. High levels of uric acid may also cause kidney stones.

URINALYSIS (u-rih-NAL-ih-sis): Examination of urine as an aid in the diagnosis of disease. Routine urinalysis involves the observation of unusual color or odor; determination of specific gravity (amount of materials dissolved in urine); chemical tests (for protein, sugar, acetone); and microscopic examination for bacteria, blood cells, and sediment. Urinalysis is used to detect abnormal functioning of the kidneys and bladder, infections, abnormal growths, and diabetes mellitus. The laboratory symbol is *UA.*

WESTERN BLOT (WES-tern blot): Test used to detect infection by *HIV* (AIDS virus). It is more specific than the ELISA. A patient's serum is mixed with purified proteins from HIV, and the reaction is examined. If the patient has made antibodies to HIV, those antibodies will react with the purified HIV proteins, and the test will be positive.

WHITE BLOOD CELL (WBC) COUNT: Determination of the number of leukocytes in the blood. Higher than normal counts can indicate the presence of infection or leukemia. A *differential* is the percentages of different types of white blood cells (neutrophils, eosinophils, basophils, lymphocytes, and monocytes) in a sample of blood. It gives more specific information about leukocytes and aids in the diagnosis of allergic diseases, disorders of the immune system, and various forms of leukemia.

ABBREVIATIONS AND SYMBOLS

ABBREVIATIONS

AB	Abortion
ABC	Aspiration, biopsy, cytology
abd	Abdomen
a.c., ac	Before meals *(ante cibum)*
ACE	Angiotensin converting enzyme (ACE inhibitors are used to treat hypertension)
ACTH	Adrenocorticotropic hormone (secreted by the pituitary gland)
AD	Right ear *(auris dexter)*
ADH	Antidiuretic hormone (secreted by the pituitary gland)
ad lib	Freely as desired *(ad libitum)*
AIDS	Acquired immunodeficiency syndrome
alb	Albumin (protein)
ALL	Acute lymphocytic leukemia
alk phos	Alkaline phosphatase (enzyme elevated in liver disease)
ALS	Amyotrophic lateral sclerosis (Lou Gehrig disease)
ALT	Alanine transaminase (enzyme elevated in liver disease); SGPT
AML	Acute myelocytic leukemia
AP	Anteroposterior (front to back)
A&P	Auscultation and percussion
aq	Water *(aqua)*
AS	Left ear *(auris sinister)*
ASD	Atrial septal defect
ASHD	Arteriosclerotic heart disease
AST	Aspartate aminotransferase (elevated in liver and heart disease); SGOT
AU	Both ears *(auris uterque)*
AV	Atrioventricular; arteriovenous
A&W	Alive and well
BaE (BE)	Barium enema
B cells	White blood cells (lymphocytes) produced in the bone marrow
b.i.d., bid	Twice a day *(bis in die)*
BM	Bowel movement; bone marrow
BMT	Bone marrow transplant
BP, B/P	Blood pressure
BPH	Benign prostatic hypertrophy
Bronch	Bronchoscopy
bs	Blood sugar; bowel sounds; breath sounds
BSE	Breast self-examination
BUN	Blood urea nitrogen (test of kidney function)
BW	Birth weight
Bx	Biopsy

c̄	With *(cum)*
C1, C2	First, second cervical vertebra
Ca	Calcium; cancer; carcinoma
CABG	Coronary artery bypass graft
CAD	Coronary artery disease
CAPD	Continuous ambulatory peritoneal dialysis
cap	Capsule
cath	Catheterize; catheterization
CBC	Complete blood count
cc	Cubic centimeter (1/1000 liter)
CC	Chief complaint
CCU	Coronary care unit
CF	Cystic fibrosis
Chemo	Chemotherapy
CHF	Congestive heart failure
Chol	Cholesterol
CIN	Cervical intra-epithelial neoplasia
CIS	Carcinoma in situ
cm	Centimeter (1/100 meter)
CML	Chronic myelocytic (myelogenous) leukemia
CNS	Central nervous system
c/o	Complains of
CO_2	Carbon dioxide
COPD	Chronic obstructive pulmonary disease
CP	Cerebral palsy; chest pain
CPD	Cephalopelvic disproportion
CPR	Cardiopulmonary resuscitation
C&S, C+S	Culture and sensitivity
CS	Cesarean section
C-section	Cesarean section
CSF	Cerebrospinal fluid
CT	Computed tomography (see CT scan)
CT (CAT) scan	Computed axial tomography (x-ray images in cross-sectional view)
CVA	Cerebrovascular accident (stroke)
c/w	Consistent with
CXR	Chest x-ray
cysto	Cystoscopy
D/C	Discontinue; discharge
D&C	Dilation and curettage (of the uterine lining)
DES	Diethylstilbestrol (estrogen causing defects in children whose mothers took the drug during pregnancy)
DJD	Degenerative joint disease
diff	Differential (percentages of types of white blood cells)

DM	Diabetes mellitus
DNA	Deoxyribonucleic acid
DOB	Date of birth
DOE	Dyspnea on exertion
DRE	Digital rectal exam
DT	Delirium tremens (caused by alcohol withdrawal)
DTR	Deep tendon reflex
DVT	Deep vein thrombosis
Dx	Diagnosis
EBV	Epstein-Barr virus (cause of mononucleosis)
ECC	Emergency cardiac care
ECG (EKG)	Electrocardiogram
Echo	Echocardiogram
ECMO	Extracorporeal membrane oxygenator
ECT	Electroconvulsive therapy
ED	Emergency department
EDC	Estimated date of confinement
EEG	Electroencephalogram
EGD	Esophagogastroduodenoscopy
ELISA	Enzyme-linked immunosorbent assay (AIDS test)
EMG	Electromyogram
ENT	Ears, nose, throat
Eos	Eosinophil (type of white blood cell)
ER	Emergency room; estrogen receptor
ERCP	Endoscopic retrograde cholangiopancreatography
ESR	Erythrocyte sedimentation rate; see sed rate
ESRD	End-stage renal disease
ESWL	Extracorporeal shock-wave lithotripsy
ETOH	Ethyl alcohol
ETT	Exercise tolerance test; endotracheal tube
FBS	Fasting blood sugar
FDA	Food and Drug Administration
Fe	Iron
FH	Family history
FHT	Fetal heart tones
FSH	Follicle-stimulating hormone (secreted by the pituitary gland)
F/U, f/u	Follow-up
5-FU	5-Fluorouracil (drug used in cancer chemotherapy)
FUO	Fever of unknown origin
Fx	Fracture
g (gm)	Gram
Ga	Gallium (element used in nuclear medicine diagnostic tests)

GB	Gallbladder
GC	Gonococcus (bacterial cause of gonorrhea)
GDM	Gestational diabetes mellitus (during pregnancy)
GERD	Gastroesophageal reflux disease
GH	Growth hormone (secreted by the pituitary gland)
GI	Gastrointestinal
Grav. 1,2	First, second pregnancy
gt, gtt	Drop, drops
GTT	Glucose tolerance test
GU	Genitourinary
Gyn	Gynecology
H	Hydrogen
h, hr	Hour
HBV	Hepatitis B virus
HCG	Human chorionic gonadotropin (secreted during pregnancy)
Hct	Hematocrit
HD	Hemodialysis (artificial kidney machine)
HDL	High-density lipoproteins (associated with decreased incidence of coronary artery disease)
HEENT	Head, ears, eyes, nose, and throat
Hg	Mercury
Hgb	Hemoglobin
HIV	Human immunodeficiency virus
h/o	History of
H_2O	Water
HPV	Human papilloma virus
HRT	Hormone replacement therapy
h.s.	At bedtime (*hora somni*)
HSG	Hysterosalpingography
HSV-1,2	Herpes simplex virus type 1, 2
HTN	Hypertension (high blood pressure)
Hx	History
I	Iodine
I&D	Incision and drainage
IBD	Inflammatory bowel disease
IBS	Inflammatory bowel syndrome
ICU	Intensive care unit
IDDM	Insulin-dependent diabetes mellitus (type I)
IM	Intramuscular
INH	Isoniazid (drug to treat tuberculosis)
I&O	Intake and output (measurement of patient's fluids)
IOL	Intraocular lens (implant)
IUD	Intrauterine device

IV	Intravenous
IVP	Intravenous pyelogram
K⁺	Potassium
kg	Kilogram (1000 grams)
KUB	Kidneys, ureters, bladder (x-ray test)
L, l	Left; liter; lower
L1, L2	First, second lumbar vertebra
LA	Left atrium
Lap	Laparotomy
lat	Lateral
LBP	Low back pain; low blood pressure
LDH	Lactate dehydrogenase (elevations associated with heart attacks)
LDL	Low-density lipoproteins (high levels associated with heart disease)
LDR	Labor, delivery, recovery
LE	Lupus erythematosus
LEEP	Loop electrosurgical excising procedure
LES	Lower esophageal sphincter
LFT	Liver function test
LKS	Liver, kidney, spleen
LLQ	Left lower quadrant (of the abdomen)
LMP	Last menstrual period
LP	Lumbar puncture
LPN	Licensed practical nurse
LTB	Laryngotracheal bronchitis
LUQ	Left upper quadrant (of the abdomen)
LV	Left ventricle
LVH	Left ventricular hypertrophy
L&W	Living and well
lymphs	Lymphocytes
lytes	Electrolytes
m	Meter
MCH	Mean corpuscular hemoglobin (amount in each red blood cell)
MCHC	Mean corpuscular hemoglobin concentration (amount per unit of blood)
MCV	Mean corpuscular volume (size of individual red blood cell)
MD, M.D.	Doctor of medicine; muscular dystrophy
mets	Metastases
mg	Milligram (1/1000 gram)
Mg	Magnesium
MH	Marital history; mental health
MI	Myocardial infarction (heart attack)

ml	Milliliter (1/1000 liter)
mm	Millimeter (1/1000 meter)
mm Hg	Millimeters of mercury (measurement of blood pressure)
mono	Monocytes (type of white blood cell)
MRA	Magnetic resonance angiography
MRI	Magnetic resonance imaging
MS	Mitral stenosis; multiple sclerosis; mental status
MSW	Medical social worker
MVP	Mitral valve prolapse
myop	Myopia (near-sightedness)
Na$^+$	Sodium
NB	Newborn
NED	No evidence of disease
NG tube	Nasogastric tube
NICU	Neonatal intensive care unit
NIDDM	Non-insulin dependent diabetes mellitus (type 2 diabetes)
NKA	No known allergies
NPO	Nothing by mouth *(nulli per os)*
NSAID	Non-steroidal anti-inflammatory drug
NSR	Normal sinus rhythm (of the heart)
NTP	Normal temperature and pressure
N+V	Nausea and vomiting
O$_2$	Oxygen
OA	Osteoarthritis
OB	Obstetrics
OD, O.D.	Right eye *(oculus dexter)*; doctor of optometry
OPD	Outpatient department
OR	Operating room
ORIF	Open reduction, internal fixation (to set a broken bone)
os	Mouth
OS	Left eye *(oculus sinister)*
OSA	Obstructive sleep apnea
OU	Each eye *(oculus uterque)*
OV	Office visit
p̄	After; following
P	Plan; posterior; pulse; phosphorus
PA	Posteroanterior (back to front); pulmonary artery
PAC	Premature atrial contraction
PaCO$_2$	Arterial pressure of carbon dioxide in the blood; also written PCO$_2$
palp	Palpable; palpation (examine by touch)
PaO$_2$	Arterial pressure of oxygen in the blood; also written PO$_2$

Pap	Papanicolaou smear (microscopic examination of cells from the cervix and vagina)
para	Paracentesis (abdominocentesis)
Para 1,2	Woman having produced one, two viable offspring; unipara, bipara
p.c., pc	After meals (*post cibum*)
PDN	Private duty nurse
PE	Physical examination
PEEP	Positive end-expiratory pressure
per	by
PERRLA	Pupils equal, round, and reactive to light and accommodation
PET	Positron emission tomography
PE tube	Pressure-equalizing tube (ventilating tube for the eardrum)
PFT	Pulmonary function test
pH	Hydrogen ion concentration (measurement of acidity or alkalinity of a solution)
PH	Past history
PI	Present illness
PID	Pelvic inflammatory disease
PKU	Phenylketonuria (test for lack of an enzyme in infants)
PM	Afternoon (*post meridian*); post mortem
PMH	Past medical history
PND	Paroxysmal nocturnal dyspnea; postnasal drip
p/o	Postoperative
p.o., po	By mouth (*per os*)
polys	Polymorphonuclear leukocytes (neutrophils)
poplit	Popliteal (behind the knee)
post-op	After operation
PP	After meals (*post prandial*); after birth (*post partum*)
PPD	Purified protein derivative (skin test for tuberculosis)
pr	Per rectum
pre-op	Before operation (preoperative)
prep	Prepare for
p.r.n.	As needed (*pro re nata*)
procto	Proctoscopy (visual examination of the anus and rectum)
pro time	Prothrombin time (test of blood clotting)
PSA	Prostate-specific antigen
pt	Patient
PT	Physical therapy; prothrombin time
PTA	Prior to admission (to hospital)
PTCA	Percutaneous transluminal coronary angioplasty (balloon angioplasty)
PTH	Parathyroid hormone
PTR	Patient to return
PTT	Partial thromboplastin time (test of blood clotting)

PVC	Premature ventricular contraction (abnormal heart rhythm)
PVD	Peripheral vascular disease
PVT	Paroxysmal ventricular tachycardia
PWB	Partial weight bearing
q	Every (*quaque*)
q.d., qd	Each day (*quaque die*)
q.h., qh	Each hour (*quaque hora*)
q2h	Each two hours (*quaque secunda hora*)
q.i.d., qid	Four times a day (*quater in die*)
q.n., qn	Each night (*quaque nox*)
q.n.s., qns	Quantity not sufficient (*quantum non satis*)
q.s., qs	Quantity sufficient (*quantum satis*)
qt	Quart
r	Right
RA	Rheumatoid arthritis; right atrium
RBC, rbc	Red blood cell count
RIA	Radioimmunoassay (minute quantities are measured)
RIND	Reversible ischemic neurologic deficit
RLQ	Right lower quadrant (of the abdomen)
R/O	Rule out
ROM	Range of motion
ROS	Review of systems
RP	Retrograde pyelogram (urogram)
RR	Recovery room; respiration rate
RRR	Regular rate and rhythm (of the heart)
RT	Radiation therapy; recreational therapy; radiologic technologist
RUQ	Right upper quadrant (of the abdomen)
RV	Right ventricle (of the heart)
Rx	Treatment (recipe)
s̄	Without (*sine*)
S1, S2	First, second sacral vertebra
S-A node	Sinoatrial node (pacemaker of the heart)
SBFT	Small bowel follow-through (x-rays of the small intestine with contrast)
sc	Subcutaneously
sed. rate	Erythrocyte sedimentation rate (time it takes red blood cells to settle out of blood)
segs	Segmented white blood cells (granulocytes)
SERM	Selective estrogen receptor modulator (tamoxifen is an example)
s.gl.	Without glasses
SGOT	See AST
SGPT	See ALT

SH	Social history: serum hepatitis
sig	Let it be labeled
SLE	Systemic lupus erythematosus
SMA	Sequential multiple analyzer (test of blood components)
SOAP	Subjective (symptoms perceived by the patient) data, Objective (exam findings) data, Assessment (evaluation of condition), Plan (goals for treatment)
SOB	Shortness of breath
S/P	Status post (previous disease condition)
SPECT	Single photon emission computed tomography
SpGr	Specific gravity
subq	Subcutaneous
SSRI	Selective serotonin reuptake inhibitor (antidepressant drug)
staph	Staphylococci (bacteria)
STAT	Immediately (*statim*)
STD	Sexually transmitted disease
strep	Streptococci (bacteria)
Sx	Symptoms; signs
sz	Seizure
T	Temperature; thoracic
T1, T2	First, second thoracic vertebra
T$_3$	Triiodothyronine (thyroid gland hormone)
T$_4$	Thyroxine (thyroid gland hormone)
T&A	Tonsillectomy and adenoidectomy
tab	Tablet
TAB	Therapeutic abortion
TAH	Total abdominal hysterectomy
TB	Tuberculosis
T cells	Lymphocytes originating in the thymus gland
TEE	Transesophageal echocardiogram
TIA	Transient ischemic attack
TENS	Transcutaneous electrical nerve stimulator
THR	Total hip replacement
t.i.d., tid	Three times a day
TLC	Total lung capacity
TM	Tympanic membrane
TNM	Tumor, nodes, metastasis (staging system for cancer)
tomos	Tomograms (x-ray images to show an organ in depth)
TPN	Total parenteral nutrition
TPR	Temperature, pulse, respiration
TSH	Thyroid-stimulating hormone (secreted by the pituitary gland)
TUR, TURP	Transurethral resection of the prostate gland
TVH	Total vaginal hysterectomy
Tx	Treatment

UA, U/A	Urinalysis
UE	Upper extremity
UGI	Upper gastrointestinal
umb	Navel (umbilical cord region)
ung	Ointment
U/O	Urine output
URI	Upper respiratory infection
US, u/s	Ultrasound
UTI	Urinary tract infection
UV	Ultraviolet
V	Vision
VA	Visual acuity
VC	Vital capacity (of lungs)
VCUG	Voiding cystourethrogram
VF	Visual field; ventricular fibrillation
VS, V/S	Vital signs
VSD	Ventricular septal defect
VSS	Vital signs stable
V tach, VT	Ventricular tachycardia (abnormal heart rhythm)
WBC, wbc	White blood cell; white blood count
WDWN	Well developed, well nourished
W/C	Wheelchair
wd	Wound
WNL	Within normal limits
WT, wt	Weight
w/u	Work-up
XRT	Radiation therapy
y/o, yr	Year(s) old

SYMBOLS

$=$	Equal	$\male$	Male	
$\neq$	Unequal	$\rightarrow$	To (in direction of)	
$+$	Positive	$>$	Greater than	
$-$	Negative	$<$	Less than	
$\uparrow$	Above, increase	$1°, 2°$	Primary, secondary to	
$\downarrow$	Below, decrease	ℨ	Dram	
$\female$	Female	℥	Ounce	

GLOSSARY OF MEDICAL TERMS

Pronunciation of each term is given with its meaning. The syllable that gets the accent is in CAPITAL LETTERS. Terms in SMALL CAPITAL LETTERS are defined elsewhere in the glossary.

ABDOMEN (AB-do-men):   space below the chest that contains organs such as the stomach, liver, intestines, and gallbladder. Also called the ABDOMINAL CAVITY, the abdomen lies between the diaphragm and the pelvis (hip bone).

ABDOMINAL (ab-DOM-i-nal):   pertaining to the abdomen.

ABDOMINAL CAVITY (ab-DOM-i-nal KAV-ih-te):   see ABDOMEN.

ABNORMAL (ab-NOR-mal):   pertaining to being away (AB-) from the norm; irregular.

ACQUIRED IMMUNODEFICIENCY SYNDROME (ah-KWI-erd im-u-no-deh-FISH-en-se SIN-drom) or AIDS: suppression or deficiency of the immune response caused by exposure to the HUMAN IMMUNODEFICIENCY VIRUS (HIV).

ACROMEGALY (ak-ro-MEG-ah-le):   enlargement of extremities as a result of thickening of the bones and soft tissues; it is caused by excessive secretion of growth hormone from the pituitary gland (after completion of puberty).

ACUTE (ah-KUT):   sharp, sudden, and intense for a short period of time.

ADENECTOMY (ad-eh-NEK-to-me):   the removal of a gland.

ADENITIS (ad-en-NI-tis):   inflammation of a gland.

ADENOCARCINOMA (ah-deh-no-kar-sih-NO-mah):   cancerous tumor derived from glandular cells.

ADENOIDECTOMY (ah-deh-noyd-EK-to-me):   removal of the ADENOIDS.

ADENOIDS (AD-eh-noidz):   enlarged lymphatic tissue in the upper part of the throat near the nasal passageways.

ADENOMA (ah-deh-NO-mah):   benign tumor of glandular cells.

ADENOPATHY (ah-deh-NOP-ah-the):   disease of glands. Often this term refers to enlargement of lymph nodes (which are not true glands, but collections of lymphatic tissue).

ADNEXA UTERI (ad-NEKS-ah U-ter-i):   accessory structures of the uterus (ovaries and fallopian tubes).

ADRENAL CORTEX (ah-DRE-nal KOR-teks):   outermost part of the adrenal gland. The adrenal cortex secretes steroid hormones such as GLUCOCORTICOIDS (cortisone).

ADRENAL GLANDS (ah-DRE-nal glanz):   two endocrine glands, each above a kidney. The adrenal glands produce hormones such as adrenalin (epinephrine) and hydrocortisone (cortisol).

ADRENALECTOMY (ah-dre-nal-EK-to-me):   removal (excision) of adrenal glands.

ADRENALIN (ah-DREN-eh-lin):   hormone secreted by the adrenal glands. It is released into the bloodstream in response to stress, such as from fear or physical injury. Also called EPINEPHRINE.

ADRENOCORTICOTROPIC HORMONE (ah-dre-no-kor-tih-ko-TROP-ic HOR-mon):   hormone secreted by the pituitary gland. It stimulates the adrenal gland (cortex or outer region) to secrete the hormone cortisone. Also called ACTH.

ADRENOPATHY (ah-dre-NOP-a-the):   disease of ADRENAL GLANDS.

AIDS: see ACQUIRED IMMUNODEFICIENCY SYNDROME.

AIR SACS (ayr-saks): thin-walled sacs within the lung. Inhaled oxygen passes into the blood from the sacs, and carbon dioxide passes out from the blood into the sacs to be exhaled.

ALBUMINURIA (al-bu-men-U-re-ah): albumin (protein) in the urine; it indicates a malfunction of the kidney.

ALKALINE PHOSPHATASE (AL-kah-line PHOS-phah-tase): an enzyme present in blood and body tissues, such as bone and liver. Elevated in diseases such as those of bone and liver. Also called alk phos.

ALLERGIST (AL-er-jist): medical doctor specializing in identifying and treating abnormal sensitivity to foreign substances such as pollen, dust, foods, and drugs.

ALOPECIA (ah-lo-PE-shah): loss of hair; baldness.

ALT: an enzyme normally found in blood and tissues, especially the liver. Also known as SGPT; elevated in liver disease.

ALVEOLAR (al-VE-o-lar): pertaining to air sacs (alveoli) within the lungs.

ALVEOLUS (al-ve-O-lus): an air sac within the lung (pl. alveoli).

ALZHEIMER DISEASE (ALTZ-hi-mer di-ZEZ): deterioration of mental capacity (irreversible dementia) marked by intellectual deterioration, disorganization of personality, and difficulties in carrying out tasks of daily living.

AMENORRHEA (a-men-o-RE-ah): absence of menstrual periods.

AMNIOCENTESIS (am-ne-o-sen-TE-sis): surgical puncture to remove fluid from the amnion (sac surrounding the developing fetus).

ANAL (A-nal): pertaining to the anus (opening of the rectum to the outside of the body).

ANALGESIC (an-al-JE-zik): medication that reduces or eliminates pain.

ANALYSIS (ah-NAL-ih-sis): separating a substance into its component parts.

ANDROGEN (AN-dro-jen): hormone that controls the development of masculine characteristics. An example is TESTOSTERONE.

ANEMIA (ah-NE-me-ah): reduced amount of oxygen to body tissues. This may result from deficiencies and abnormalities of red blood cells or loss of blood. Literally, *anemia* means "lacking" (AN-) in "blood" (-EMIA).

ANEMIC (ah-NE-mik): pertaining to ANEMIA.

ANESTHESIOLOGIST (an-es-the-ze-OL-o-jist): medical doctor specializing in administering agents capable of bringing about loss of sensation and consciousness.

ANESTHESIOLOGY (an-es-the-ze-OL-o-je): study of how to administer agents capable of bringing about loss of sensation and consciousness.

ANEURYSM (AN-u-rizm): localized widening of the wall of an artery, vein, or of the heart. From ANA- meaning "throughout" and -EURUS meaning "wide."

ANGINA (an-JI-nah): sharp pain in the chest resulting from a decrease in blood supply to heart muscle. Also called angina pectoris (chest).

ANGINA PECTORIS (an-JI-nah PEK-tor-is): Chest pain caused by decreased blood flow to heart muscle.

ANGIOGRAPHY (an-je-OG-rah-fe): x-ray recording of blood vessels after contrast is injected.

ANGIOPLASTY (AN-je-o-plas-te): surgical repair of a blood vessel. A tube (catheter) is placed in a clogged artery and a balloon at the end of the tube is inflated to flatten the clogged material against the wall of the artery. This enlarges the opening of the artery so that more blood can pass through. Also called balloon angioplasty.

ANGIOTENSIN (AN-je-o-TEN-sin):   hormone that is a powerful vasoconstrictor and raises blood pressure.

ANKYLOSING SPONDYLITIS (ang-ki-LO-sing spon-dih-LI-tis):   chronic inflammation of the vertebrae (backbones) with stiffening of spinal joints so that movement becomes increasingly painful.

ANKYLOSIS (ang-ki-LO-sis):   stiffening and immobility of a joint caused by injury, disease, or a surgical procedure.

ANOMALY (an-NOM-ah-le):   irregularity; a deviation from the normal. A congenital anomaly (irregularity) is present at birth.

ANTE MORTEM (AN-te MOR-tem):   before death.

ANTE NATAL (AN-te NA-tal):   before birth.

ANTE PARTUM (AN-te PAR-tum):   before birth.

ANTERIOR (an-TE-re-or):   located in the front (of the body or of a structure).

ANTIANDROGEN (an-tih-AN-dro-jen):   substance that inhibits the effects of androgens (male hormones).

ANTIARRHYTHMIC (an-te-ah-RITH-mik):   pertaining to a drug that works against or prevents abnormal heartbeats (arrhythmias).

ANTIBIOTIC (an-tih-bi-OT-ik):   pertaining to a substance that works against germ or bacterial life.

ANTIBODY (AN-tih-bod-e):   a substance that works against (ANTI-) germs ("bodies" of infection). Antibodies are produced by white blood cells when germs (antigens) enter the bloodstream.

ANTICOAGULANT (an-tih-ko-AG-u-lant):   drug that prevents clotting (coagulation). Anticoagulants are given when there is danger of clots forming in blood vessels.

ANTICONVULSANT (an-tih-kon-VULS-ent):   drug that prevents or relieves convulsions (involuntary muscular contractions).

ANTIDEPRESSANT (an-tih-de-PRES-ent):   drug used to prevent or treat depression.

ANTIDIABETIC (an-tih-di-ah-BET-ik):   drug that prevents or relieves symptoms of diabetes.

ANTIESTROGEN (an-tih-ES-tro-jen):   substance that inhibits the effects of estrogens (female hormones).

ANTIFUNGAL (an-tih-FUNG-al):   drug that destroys or inhibits the growth of fungi (organisms such as yeasts, molds, and mushrooms).

ANTIGEN (AN-tih-jen):   foreign agent (germ) that stimulates white blood cells to make antibodies. Antigens are then destroyed by the antibodies.

ANTIHISTAMINE (an-tih-HIS-tah-men):   drug used to counteract the effects of histamine production in allergic reactions and colds.

ANTIHYPERTENSIVE (an-ti-hi-per-TEN-siv):   drug that reduces high blood pressure.

ANTITUBERCULAR (an-tih-too-BER-ku-lar):   an agent or drug used to treat tuberculosis.

ANTIVIRAL (an-tih-VI-ral):   agent that inhibits and prevents the growth and reproduction of viruses.

ANURIA (an-U-re-ah):   lack of urine formation by the kidney.

ANUS (A-nus):   opening of the rectum to the surface of the body; solid wastes (feces) leave the body through the anus.

AORTA (a-OR-tah):   largest artery, which leads from the lower left chamber of the heart to arteries all over the body.

AORTIC STENOSIS (a-OR-tik steh-NO-sis):   narrowing of the aorta.

APEX (A-peks):   pointed end of an organ (pl. apices [A-pih-sez]).

APHAKIA (ah-FA-ke-ah):   absence of the lens of the eye.

APHASIA (ah-FA-ze-ah):   absence or impairment of communication through speech.

APNEA (AP-ne-ah):   not (A-) able to breathe (-PNEA).

APPENDECTOMY (ap-en-DEK-to-me):   removal of the appendix.

APPENDICITIS (ap-en-dih-SI-tis):   inflammation of the appendix.

APPENDIX (ah-PEN-dikz):   small sac that hangs from the juncture of the small and large intestines in the right lower quadrant of the abdomen. Its function is unknown.

AREOLA (ah-RE-o-lah):   dark, pigmented area around the nipple of the breast.

ARRHYTHMIA (a-RITH-me-ah):   abnormal heart rhythm.

ARTERIOGRAPHY (ar-ter-e-OG-ra-fe):   process of recording (x-ray) of arteries after injecting contrast material.

ARTERIOLE (ar-TER-e-ol):   small artery.

ARTERIOLITIS (ar-ter-e-o-LI-tis):   inflammation of small arteries (arterioles).

ARTERIOSCLEROSIS (ar-ter-e-o-skle-RO-sis):   hardening of arteries. The most common form is *atherosclerosis,* which is hardening of arteries caused by collection of fatty, cholesterol-like deposits (plaque) in arteries.

ARTERY (AR-ter-e):   largest blood vessel. Arteries carry blood away from the heart.

ARTHRALGIA (ar-THRAL-je-ah):   pain in a joint.

ARTHRITIS (ar-THRI-tis):   inflammation of a joint.

ARTHROCENTESIS (ar-thro-sen-TE-sis):   surgical puncture to remove fluid from a joint.

ARTHROGRAM (AR-thro-gram):   x-ray record of a joint.

ARTHROPATHY (ar-THROP-ah-the):   disease of joints.

ARTHROSCOPE (AR-thro-skop):   instrument used to examine the inside of a joint.

ARTHROSCOPY (ar-THROS-ko-pe):   process of visual examination of a joint.

ARTHROSIS (ar-THRO-sis):   abnormal condition of a joint.

ASCITES (ah-SI-tez):   abnormal collection of fluid in the abdomen.

ASPHYXIA (as-FIK-se-ah):   deficiency of oxygen in the blood and increase in carbon dioxide in blood and tissues. Major symptom is a complete absence of breathing.

AST: an enzyme normally present in blood and tissues such as heart and liver. Also called SGOT.

ASTHMA (AZ-mah):   difficult breathing caused by a spasm of the bronchial tubes or a swelling of their mucous membrane lining.

ATELECTASIS (ah-teh-LEK-tah-sis):   collapsed lung (ATEL- meaning "incomplete"; -ECTASIS meaning "widening or dilation").

ATHEROSCLEROSIS (ah-theh-ro-skle-RO-sis):   see ARTERIOSCLEROSIS.

ATRIUM (A-tre-um):   upper chamber of the heart (pl. atria).

ATROPHY (AT-ro-fe):   decrease in size of cells within an organ.

AUDITORY CANAL (AW-dih-to-re kah-NAL):   passageway leading into the ear from the outside of the body.

AUDITORY NERVE (AW-dih-to-re nurve): nerve that carries messages from the inner ear to the brain, making hearing possible.

AURA (AW-rah): a strange sensation coming before more definite symptoms of illness. An aura often precedes a migraine headache, warning the patient that an attack is beginning.

AURAL DISCHARGE (AW-rah DIS-charge): fluid or material from the ear.

AUTOPSY (AW-top-se): examination of a dead body to discover the actual cause of death. Also called a post mortem exam or necropsy. Literally, it means "to see" (-OPSY) with "one's own" (AUTO-) eyes.

AXIAL (AKS-e-al): pertaining to an axis (a line through the center of a body or about which a structure revolves).

AXILLARY (AKS-ih-lar-e): pertaining to the armpit or underarm.

BACTERICIDAL (bak-tih-re-SI-dal): pertaining to an agent that destroys bacteria.

BACTERIOSTATIC (bak-tih-re-o-STAT-ik): pertaining to an agent that inhibits bacterial growth.

BACTERIUM (bak-TIH-re-um): type of one-celled organism whose genetic material (DNA) is not organized within a nucleus (pl. bacteria).

BALANITIS (bah-lah-NI-tis): inflammation of the penis.

BARIUM (BAH-re-um): substance used as an opaque (x-rays cannot pass through it) contrast medium for x-ray examination of the digestive tract.

BARIUM ENEMA (BAH-re-um EN-eh-mah): x-ray image of the lower digestive tract after injection of a solution of barium into the rectum.

BARIUM MEAL (SWALLOW) (BAH-re-um mel): x-ray image of the upper digestive tract after the patient swallows a solution of barium.

BENIGN (be-NIN): not cancerous; a tumor that does not spread and is limited in growth.

BENIGN PROSTATIC HYPERPLASIA (be-NIN pro-STAH-tik hi-per-PLA-ze-ah): non-malignant enlargement of the prostate gland.

BENZODIAZEPINE (be-zo-di-AZ-eh-pin): drug used to relieve anxiety, relax muscles, and produce sedation.

BETA BLOCKER (BAY-tah BLOK-er): drug that is used for the treatment of high blood pressure (hypertension), chest pain (angina), and abnormal rhythms of the heart (arrhythmias).

BILATERAL (bi-LAT-er-al): pertaining to two (both) sides.

BILE (bil): a yellow or orange fluid produced by the liver. It breaks up large fat globules and helps the digestion of fats.

BILE DUCT (bil dukt): tube that carries bile from the liver and gallbladder to the intestine.

BILIRUBIN (bil-ih-RU-bin): a red blood cell pigment excreted with bile from the liver into the intestine.

BIOLOGY (bi-OL-o-je): study of life.

BIOPSY (BI-op-se): process of viewing living tissue under a microscope.

BLADDER (BLAD-der): see URINARY BLADDER.

BONE (bon): hard, rigid type of connective tissue that makes up most of the skeleton. It is composed of calcium salts.

BONE MARROW (bon MAH-ro):   soft, sponge-like material in the inner part of bones. Blood cells are made in the bone marrow.

BRADYCARDIA (bra-de-KAR-de-ah):   slow heartbeat.

BRAIN (bran):   organ in the head that controls the activities of the body.

BREAST (brest):   one of two glandular organs in front of the chest. The breasts produce milk after childbirth.

BRONCHIAL TUBE (BRONG-ke-al tube):   one of two tubes that carry air from the windpipe to the lungs. Also called a bronchus (pl. bronchi).

BRONCHIOLE (BRONG-ke-OL):   small bronchial tube.

BRONCHIOLITIS (brong-ke-o-LI-tis):   inflammation of bronchioles.

BRONCHITIS (brong-KI-tis):   inflammation of bronchial tubes.

BRONCHOSCOPE (BRONG-ko-skop):   instrument used to visually examine bronchial tubes.

BRONCHOSCOPY (brong-KOS-ko-pe):   visual examination of bronchial tubes by passing an endoscope through the trachea (windpipe) into the bronchi.

BRONCHUS (BRONG-kus):   see BRONCHIAL TUBE.

BURSA (BUR-sah):   sac of fluid near a joint (pl. bursae [BUR-see]).

BURSITIS (bur-SI-tis):   inflammation of a bursa.

CALCANEUS (kal-KA-ne-us):   heel bone.

CALCIUM CHANNEL BLOCKER (KAL-se-um CHA-nal BLOK-er):   drug that dilates arteries by inhibiting the flow of calcium into muscle cells that line arteries. It is used to treat hypertension (high blood pressure) and angina (chest pain caused by insufficient oxygen to heart muscle).

CALCULUS (KAL-ku-lus):   stone (pl. calculi [KAL-ku-li]).

CAPILLARY (KAP-il-lar-e):   smallest blood vessel (pl. capillaries).

CARBON DIOXIDE (KAHR-bon di-OK-side):   odorless, colorless gas formed in tissues and eliminated by the lungs.

CARCINOMA (kar-sih-NO-mah):   cancerous tumor. Carcinomas form from epithelial cells, which line the internal organs as well as cover the outside of the body.

CARDIAC (KAR-de-ak):   pertaining to the heart.

CARDIOLOGIST (kar-de-OL-o-jist):   physician specializing in the study of the heart and heart disease.

CARDIOLOGY (kar-de-OL-o-je):   study of the heart.

CARDIOMEGALY (kar-de-o-MEG-ah-le):   enlargement of the heart.

CARDIOMYOPATHY (kar-de-o-mi-OP-ah-the):   disease of heart muscle.

CARDIOVASCULAR SURGEON (kar-de-o-VAS-ku-lar SUR-jin):   specialist in operating on the heart and blood vessels.

CARDIOVERSION (KAR-de-o-ver-zhun):   brief discharges of electricity passing across the chest to stop a cardiac ARRHYTHMIA. Also called defibrillation.

CARPALS (KAR-palz):   wrist bones.

CARPAL TUNNEL SYNDROME (KAR-pal TUN-el SIN-drom):   group of symptoms resulting from compression of the median nerve in the wrist. Symptoms include tingling, pain, and burning sensations in the hand and wrist.

CARTILAGE (KAR-tih-lij):   flexible, fibrous connective tissue, found attached to the nose, ears, voice box, and windpipe, and chiefly attached to bones at joints.

CATARACT (KAT-ah-raht):   clouding of the lens of the eye.

CATHARTIC (ka-THAR-tik):   pertaining to a substance that causes the release of feces from the large intestine.

CAT SCAN (kat scan):   computerized axial tomography. See CT SCAN.

CELL (sel):   smallest unit or part of an organ.

CELLULITIS (sel-u-LI-tis):   inflammation of soft tissue under the skin; it is marked by swelling, redness, and pain and is caused by bacterial infection.

CEPHALGIA (seh-FAL-je-ah):   headache. Shortened form of cephalalgia.

CEPHALIC (seh-FAL-ik):   pertaining to the head.

CEPHALOSPORIN (sef-ah-lo-SPOR-in):   antibiotic similar to penicillin and used to treat infections of the respiratory tract, ear, urinary tract, bones, and blood.

CEREBELLAR (ser-eh-BEL-ar):   pertaining to the cerebellum.

CEREBELLUM (ser-eh-BEL-um):   lower, back part of the brain that coordinates muscle movement and balance.

CEREBRAL (seh-RE-bral or SER-e-bral):   pertaining to the CEREBRUM.

CEREBROVASCULAR ACCIDENT (seh-re-bro-VAS-ku-lar AK-sih-dent): disorder of blood vessels within the cerebrum. It results from inadequate blood supply to the brain. See also STROKE.

CEREBRUM (seh-RE-brum):   largest part of the brain. It controls thought processes, hearing, speech, vision, and body movements.

CERVICAL (SER-vi-kal):   pertaining to the neck of the body or the neck (cervix) of the uterus.

CERVICAL REGION (SER-vi-kal RE-jin):   seven backbones in the area of the neck.

CERVICAL VERTEBRA (SER-vi-kal VER-teh-brah):   backbone in the neck.

CERVIX (SER-viks):   lower, neck-like portion of the uterus opening into the vagina.

CESAREAN SECTION (seh-ZAR-re-an SEK-shun):   incision of the uterus to remove the fetus at birth.

CHEMOTHERAPY (ke-mo-THER-ah-pe):   treatment with drugs. Chemotherapy is most often used in the treatment for cancer.

CHOLECYSTECTOMY (ko-le-sis-TEK-to-me):   removal of the gallbladder.

CHOLEDOCHODUODENOSTOMY (ko-led-oh-ko-doo-o-deh-NOS-to-me):   new surgical attachment of the common bile duct to the duodenum.

CHOLEDOCHOTOMY (ko-led-o-KOT-o-me):   incision of the common bile duct.

CHOLELITHIASIS (ko-le-lih-THI-ah-sis):   abnormal condition of gallstones.

CHOLESTEROL (ko-LES-ter-ol):   substance made in the liver and found in the bloodstream. It is an important part of cells and is necessary for creating hormones. It may accumulate in the lining of arteries, such as in the heart, causing heart disease.

CHONDROMA (kon-DRO-mah):   benign tumor of cartilage.

CHONDROSARCOMA (kon-dro-sar-KO-mah):   malignant tumor of CARTILAGE.

CHRONIC (KRON-ik):   lasting a long time.

CHRONIC OBSTRUCTIVE PULMONARY DISEASE (KRON-ik ob-STRUK-tiv PUL-mo-na-re DEH-zes):   chronic limitation in airflow into and out of the body; includes chronic bronchitis, ASTHMA, and EMPHYSEMA.

CIRCULATORY SYSTEM (SER-ku-lah-tor-e SIS-tem):   organs (heart and blood vessels) that carry blood throughout the body.

CIRRHOSIS (seh-RO-sis):   liver disease with deterioration of the liver cells. Cirrhosis is often caused by alcoholism and poor nutrition.

CLAVICLE (KLAV-ih-kuhl):   collar bone.

CLINICAL (KLIN-eh-kal):   pertaining to the bedside or clinic; involving patient care.

COCCYGEAL (kok-sih-JE-al):   pertaining to the tailbone (coccyx).

COCCYGEAL REGION (kok-sih-JE-al RE-jin):   four fused (joined together) bones at the base of the spinal column (backbone).

COCCYX (KOK-siks):   tailbone.

COLECTOMY (ko-LEK-to-me):   removal of the colon (large intestine).

COLITIS (ko-LI-tis):   inflammation of the colon (large intestine).

COLON (KO-lon):   large intestine (bowel).

COLONIC POLYPOSIS (ko-LON-ik pol-ih-PO-sis):   growths or masses protruding from the mucous membrane lining the colon.

COLONOSCOPY (ko-lon-OS-ko-pe):   visual examination of the colon.

COLORECTAL SURGEON (ko-lo-REK-tal SUR-jin):   physician specializing in operating on the colon and rectum.

COLOSTOMY (ko-LOS-to-me):   opening of the colon to the outside of the body.

COLPOSCOPY (kol-POS-ko-pe):   visual examination of the vagina and cervix.

CONCUSSION (kon-KUS-un):   loss of consciousness resulting from a blow to the head.

CONGENITAL ANOMALY (con-JEN-ih-tal ah-NOM-ah-le):   see ANOMALY.

CONGESTIVE HEART FAILURE (kon-JES-tiv hart FAIL-ur):   condition in which the heart is unable to pump its required amount of blood, resulting in inadequate oxygen to body cells.

CONIZATION (ko-nih-ZA-shun):   removal of a wedge-shaped piece (cone) of tissue from the cervix in the diagnosis and treatment of early cancer of the cervix.

CONJUNCTIVA (kon-junk-TI-vah):   thin protective membrane over the front of the eye and attached to the eyelids.

CONJUNCTIVITIS (kon-junk-ti-VI-tis):   inflammation of the CONJUNCTIVA.

CONNECTIVE TISSUE (kon-NEK-tiv TIS-u):   fibrous tissue that supports and connects internal organs, bones, and walls of blood vessels.

CORIUM (KOR-e-um):   middle layer of the skin below the epidermis; DERMIS.

CORNEA (KOR-ne-ah):   transparent layer over the front of the eye. It bends light to focus it on sensitive cells (retina) at the back of the eye.

CORONAL PLANE (kor-O-nal playn):   see FRONTAL PLANE.

CORONARY (KOR-on-ary):   pertaining to the heart.

CORONARY ARTERIES (KOR-on-ary AR-ter-ez):   blood vessels that carry oxygen-rich blood from the AORTA to the heart muscle.

CORTEX (KOR-teks):   outer part of an organ (pl. cortices [KOR-teh-sez]).

CORTISOL (KOR-tih-sol):   anti-inflammatory hormone secreted by the adrenal cortex.

COSTOCHONDRITIS (kos-to-kon-DRI-tis):   inflammation of a rib and its cartilage.

COSTOCHONDRAL (kos-to-KON-dral):   pertaining to a rib and its cartilage.

CRANIAL CAVITY (KRA-ne-al KAV-ih-te):   space surrounded by the skull and containing the brain and other organs.

CRANIOTOMY (kra-ne-OT-o-me):   incision of the skull.

CRANIUM (KRA-ne-um): skull.

CREATININE (kre-AT-tih-nin): nitrogen-containing waste that is removed from the blood by the kidney and excreted in urine.

CROHN DISEASE (kron dih-zes): inflammation of the gastrointestinal tract (often the ILEUM) marked by bouts of diarrhea, abdominal cramping, and fever. Along with ulcerative colitis, Crohn disease is a type of INFLAMMATORY BOWEL DISEASE.

CROSS SECTION (kros SEK-shun): divides an organ or the body into upper and lower portions; TRANSVERSE PLANE.

CRYOTHERAPY (kri-o-THER-ah-pe): treatment using cold (CRY/O-) temperatures.

CRYPTORCHISM (kript-OR-kism): undescended (CRYPT- means "hidden") testicle. The testicle is not in the scrotal sac at birth.

CT SCAN: computed tomography; series of x-ray images showing organs in cross-section (transverse view). Also called a CAT SCAN.

CUSHING SYNDROME (KOOSH-ing SIN-drom): symptoms produced by an excess of cortisol from the adrenal cortex. Cushing syndrome is marked by moon face, fatty swellings, and weakness.

CYANOSIS (si-ah-NO-sis): bluish discoloration of the skin due to deficient OXYGEN in the bloodstream.

CYSTITIS (sis-TI-tis): inflammation of the urinary bladder.

CYSTOSCOPE (SIS-to-skop): instrument (endoscope) used to view the urinary bladder.

CYSTOSCOPY (sis-TOS-ko-pe): visual examination of the urinary bladder.

CYTOLOGY (si-TOL-o-je): study of cells.

DEBRIDEMENT (de-BREED-ment): removal of diseased tissue from the skin.

DEFIBRILLATION (de-fib-rih-LA-shun): brief discharges of electricity applied to the chest to stop an abnormal heart rhythm.

DEMENTIA (deh-MEN-shah): loss of memory and mental abilities.

DERMAL (DER-mal): pertaining to the skin.

DERMATITIS (der-mah-TI-tis): inflammation of the skin.

DERMATOLOGIST (der-mah-TOL-o-jist): physician specializing in the skin and its diseases.

DERMATOLOGY (der-mah-TOL-o-je): study of the skin and its diseases.

DERMATOSIS (der-mah-TO-sis): any abnormal condition of the skin.

DERMIS (DER-mis): fibrous middle layer of the skin below the epidermis. The dermis contains nerves and blood vessels, hair roots, oil and sweat glands; the CORIUM.

DIABETES MELLITUS (di-ah-BE-tez MEL-li-tus): disorder marked by deficient INSULIN in the blood, which causes sugar to remain in the blood rather than entering cells. Diabetes is named from a Greek word meaning "siphon" (through which water passes easily). One symptom is frequent urination (polyuria). Type 1 diabetes is marked by lack of insulin, and patients require injections of insulin. In Type 2 diabetes, insulin is not adequately or appropriately secreted. Type 2 diabetes has a tendency to develop later in life, and patients are treated with diet, exercise, and oral antidiabetic drugs.

DIAGNOSIS (di-ag-NO-sis): complete knowledge of patient's condition (pl. diagnoses).

DIALYSIS (di-AL-ih-sis): complete separation (-LYSIS) of wastes (urea) from the blood when the kidneys fail. See also HEMODIALYSIS and PERITONEAL DIALYSIS.

DIAPHRAGM (DI-ah-fram): muscle that separates the chest from the abdomen.

DIARRHEA (di-ah-RE-ah): discharge of watery wastes from the COLON.

DIGESTIVE SYSTEM (di-JES-tiv SIS-tem): organs that bring food into the body and break it down to enter the bloodstream or eliminate it through the rectum and anus.

DILATION (di-LA-shun): widening; dilatation.

DILATION AND CURETTAGE (di-LA-shun and kur-ih-TAJ): widening of the opening to the cervix and scraping (curettage) of the inner lining of the uterus; *D&C.*

DISC (DISK): piece of cartilage that is between each backbone.

DIURETIC (di-u-RET-ik): drug that causes kidneys to allow more fluid (as urine) to leave the body. Diuretics are used to treat HYPERTENSION. DI- (from DIA-) means "complete," and UR- means "urine."

DIVERTICULA (di-ver-TIK-u-lah): small pouches or sacs created by herniation of mucous membrane linings, often in the intestines (sing. diverticulum).

DIVERTICULOSIS (di-ver-tik-u-LO-sis): abnormal condition of small pouches in the lining of the intestines.

DUODENAL (do-o-DE-nal): pertaining to the duodenum.

DUODENUM (do-o-DE-num): first part of the small intestine.

DYSENTERY (DIS-en-the-re): painful intestines.

DYSMENORRHEA (dis-men-o-RE-ah): painful menstrual flow.

DYSPEPSIA (dis-PEP-se-ah): painful (DYS-) digestion (-PEPSIA).

DYSPHAGIA (dis-FA-jah): difficult swallowing.

DYSPHASIA (dis-FA-zhah): difficult (impairment of) speech.

DYSPLASIA (dis-PLA-zhah): abnormality of the development or the formation of cells. Normal cells change in size, shape, and organization.

DYSPNEA (disp-NE-ah): painful (DYS-) (labored, difficult) breathing (-PNEA).

DYSURIA (dis-U-re-ah): painful or difficult urination.

EAR: organ that receives sound waves and transmits them to nerves leading to the brain.

EARDRUM (EAR-drum): membrane separating the outer and middle parts of the ear; the tympanic membrane.

ECTOPIC PREGNANCY (ek-TOP-ik PREG-nan-se): development of the fetus in a place other than the uterus. The fallopian tubes are the most common ectopic site.

EDEMA (eh-DE-mah): swelling in tissues. Edema is often caused by retention (holding back) of fluid and salt by the kidneys.

ELECTROCARDIOGRAM (e-lek-tro-KAR-de-o-gram): record of the electricity in the heart.

ELECTROENCEPHALOGRAM (e-lek-tro-en-SEF-ah-lo-gram): record of the electricity in the brain.

ELECTROENCEPHALOGRAPHY (e-lek-tro-en-sef-ah-LOG-ra-fe): process of recording the electricity in the brain.

ELECTROLYTE (eh-LEK-tro-lite):   substance (calcium, potassium, sodium) that conducts an electric current and is found in blood (serum) and body cells.

EMBRYO (EM-bre-o):   a new organism in the earliest stage of development. At the end of the second month of pregnancy, the developing baby is called a FETUS.

EMERGENCY MEDICINE (e-MER-jen-se MED-ih-sin):   care of patients requiring immediate action.

EMPHYSEMA (em-fih-SE-mah):   lung disorder in which air becomes trapped in the air sacs and bronchioles, making breathing difficult. Emphysema is marked by the accumulation of mucus and the loss of elasticity in lung tissue.

ENCEPHALITIS (en-sef-ah-LI-tis):   inflammation of the brain.

ENCEPHALOPATHY (en-sef-ah-LOP-ah-the):   disease of the brain.

ENDOCARDITIS (EN-do-kar-DI-tis):   inflammation of the inner lining of the heart (endocardium).

ENDOCRINE GLANDS (EN-do-krin glanz):   organs that produce (secrete) hormones.

ENDOCRINE SYSTEM (EN-do-krin SIS-tem):   endocrine glands. Examples are the pituitary, thyroid, and adrenal glands and the pancreas.

ENDOCRINOLOGIST (en-do-krih-NOL-o-jist):   specialist in the study of endocrine glands and their disorders.

ENDOCRINOLOGY (en-do-krih-NOL-o-je):   study of ENDOCRINE GLANDS.

ENDOMETRIOSIS (en-do-me-tre-O-sis):   an abnormal condition in which tissue from the inner lining of the uterus is found outside the uterus, usually in the pelvic cavity.

ENDOMETRIUM (en-do-ME-tre-um):   inner lining of the uterus.

ENDOSCOPE (EN-do-skop):   instrument used to view a hollow organ or body cavity; a tube fitted with a lens system that allows viewing in different directions.

ENDOSCOPIC RETROGRADE CHOLANGIOPANCREATOGRAPHY (en-do-SKOP-ik RET-tro-grade kol-an-je-o-pan-kre-ah-TOG-rah-fe):   x-ray images of bile ducts and pancreas after injecting contrast through a catheter from the mouth, esophagus, and stomach into bile and pancreatic ducts.

ENDOSCOPY (en-DOS-ko-pe):   process of viewing the inside of hollow organs or cavities by using an endoscope.

ENTERIC (en-TER-ik):   pertaining to the small intestine.

ENTERITIS (en-teh-RI-tis):   inflammation of the small intestine.

EPIDERMIS (ep-i-DER-mis):   outer (EPI-) layer of the skin (-DERMIS).

EPIDURAL HEMATOMA (ep-ih-DUR-al he-mah-TO-mah):   mass of blood above the dura mater (outermost layer of membranes surrounding the brain and spinal cord).

EPIGLOTTIS (ep-ih-GLOT-tis):   flap of cartilage that covers the mouth of the trachea when swallowing occurs so that food cannot enter the airway.

EPIGLOTTITIS (ep-ih-glo-TI-tis):   inflammation of the EPIGLOTTIS.

EPILEPSY (ep-ih-LEP-se):   condition in which abnormal electrical activity in the brain results in sudden, fleeting disturbances in nerve cell functioning. An attack of epilepsy is called a SEIZURE.

EPINEPHRINE (eh-pih-NEF-rin):   hormone secreted by the adrenal gland in response to stress and physical injury. It is a drug used to treat hypersensitivity reactions (severe allergy), asthma, bronchial spasm, and nasal congestion. Also called ADRENALIN.

EPITHELIAL (ep-ih-THE-le-al): pertaining to skin cells. This term originally described cells on (EPI-) the breast nipple (THELI-). Now, it indicates all cells lining the inner part of internal organs as well as covering the outside of the body.

ERYTHROCYTE (eh-RITH-ro-site): red blood cell.

ERYTHROCYTOSIS (eh-rith-ro-si-TO-sis): abnormal condition (slight increase in numbers) of red blood cells.

ERYTHROMYCIN (eh-rith-ro-MI-sin): an antibiotic that is produced from a red (ERYTHR/O-) mold (-MYCIN).

ESOPHAGEAL (eh-sof-ah-JE-al): pertaining to the esophagus.

ESOPHAGITIS (eh-sof-ah-JI-tis): inflammation of the esophagus.

ESOPHAGOSCOPY (eh-sof-ah-GOS-ko-pe): visual examination of the esophagus.

ESOPHAGUS (eh-SOF-ah-gus): tube leading from the throat to the stomach.

ESTROGEN (ES-tro-jen): hormone that promotes the development of female secondary sex characteristics. Examples are estradiol, estriol, and conjugated estrogen.

EUSTACHIAN TUBE (u-STA-she-an tub): channel connecting the middle part of the ear with the throat.

EXCISION (ek-SIZH-un): act of cutting out, removing, or resecting.

EXOCRINE GLANDS (EK-so-krin glanz): glands that produce (secrete) chemicals that leave the body through tubes (ducts). Examples are tear, sweat, and salivary glands.

EXOPHTHALMIC GOITER (ek-sof-THAL-mik GOY-ter): enlargement of the thyroid gland accompanied by high levels of thyroid hormone in the blood and protrusion of the eyeballs (EXOPHTHALMOS).

EXOPHTHALMOS (ek-sof-THAL-mos): abnormal protrusion of eyeballs usually caused by HYPERTHYROIDISM.

EXTRACRANIAL (eks-tra-KRA-ne-al): pertaining to outside the skull.

EXTRAHEPATIC (eks-tra-heh-PAT-ik): pertaining to outside the liver.

EXTRAPULMONARY (eks-trah-PUL-mo-nah-re): outside the lungs.

EYE (i): organ that receives light waves and transmits them to the brain.

FALLOPIAN TUBES (fah-LO-pe-an tubz): two tubes that lead from the ovaries to the uterus. They transport egg cells to the uterus; also called uterine tubes.

FAMILY MEDICINE (FAM-i-le MED-ih-sin): primary care of all members of the family on a continuing basis.

FAMILY PRACTITIONER (FAM-ih-le prak-TIH-shan-er): doctor responsible for primary care and treatment of patients on a continuing basis.

FELLOWSHIP TRAINING (FEL-o-ship TRA-ning): postgraduate training for doctors in specialized fields. The training may include CLINICAL and RESEARCH (laboratory) work.

FEMALE REPRODUCTIVE SYSTEM (FE-mal re-pro-DUK-tiv SIS-tem): organs that produce (OVARY) and transport (FALLOPIAN TUBES) egg cells and secrete female hormones (ESTROGEN and PROGESTERONE). The system includes the UTERUS, where the embryo and fetus grow.

FEMUR (FE-mer): thigh bone.

FETUS (FE-tus): unborn infant in the uterus after the second month of pregnancy.

FIBRILLATION (fih-brih-LA-shun):   rapid, irregular, involuntary muscular contraction. Atrial and ventricular fibrillation are cardiac (heart) ARRHYTHMIAS.

FIBROID (FI-broyd):   benign growth of muscle tissue in the uterus.

FIBROSARCOMA (fi-bro-sar-KO-mah):   malignant tumor of fibrous tissue.

FIBULA (FIB-u-lah):   smaller lower leg bone.

FIXATION (fik-SA-shun):   act of holding, sewing, or fastening a part in a fixed position.

FLUTTER (FLUT-er):   rapid but regular, abnormal heart muscle contraction. Atrial and ventricular flutter are heart ARRHYTHMIAS.

FOLLICLE-STIMULATING HORMONE (FOL-eh-kle STIM-u-la-ting HOR-mon):   a hormone secreted by the pituitary gland to stimulate the egg cells in the ovaries.

FRACTURE (FRAK-tur):   breaking of a bone.

FRONTAL (FRUN-tal):   pertaining to the front; anterior.

FRONTAL PLANE (FRUN-tal plan):   imaginary line that divides an organ or the body into a front and back portion; the coronal plane.

GALLBLADDER (GAWL-bla-der):   sac below the liver that stores bile and delivers it to the small intestine.

GANGLION (GANG-le-on):   benign cyst near a joint (wrist); also, a group of nerve cells (pl. ganglia [GANG-le-ah]).

GASTRALGIA (gas-TRAL-jah):   stomach pain.

GASTRECTOMY (gas-TREK-to-me):   excision (removal) of the stomach.

GASTRIC (GAS-trik):   pertaining to the stomach.

GASTRITIS (gas-TRI-tis):   inflammation of the stomach.

GASTROENTERITIS (gas-tro-en-teh-RI-tis):   inflammation of the stomach and intestines.

GASTROENTEROLOGIST (gas-tro-en-ter-OL-o-jist):   specialist in the treatment of stomach and intestinal disorders.

GASTROENTEROLOGY (gas-tro-en-ter-OL-o-je):   study of the stomach and intestines.

GASTROESOPHAGEAL REFLUX DISEASE (gas-tro-eh-sof-ah-JE-al RE-flux dih-zez):   backflow of contents of the stomach into the esophagus. Abbreviation is GERD.

GASTROJEJUNOSTOMY (gas-tro-jeh-ju-NOS-to-me):   new surgical opening between the stomach and the jejunum (second part of the small intestine). This procedure is also known as an anastomosis.

GASTROSCOPE (GAS-tro-skop):   instrument used to view the stomach. It is passed down the throat and esophagus into the stomach.

GASTROSCOPY (gas-TROS-ko-pe):   visual examination of the stomach.

GASTROTOMY (gas-TROT-o-me):   incision of the stomach.

GERD: see GASTROESOPHAGEAL REFLUX DISEASE

GERIATRIC (jer-e-AH-trik):   pertaining to treatment of older people.

GERIATRICIAN (jer-e-ah-TRISH-an):   specialist in the treatment of diseases of old age.

GERIATRICS (jer-e-AH-triks):   treatment of disorders of old age.

GLAND: group of cells that secretes chemicals to the outside of the body (EXOCRINE GLANDS) or directly into the bloodstream (ENDOCRINE GLANDS).

GLAUCOMA (glaw-KO-mah): increase of fluid pressure within the eye. Fluid is formed more rapidly than it is removed. The increased pressure damages sensitive cells in the back of the eye, and vision is disturbed.

GLIOBLASTOMA (gli-o-blas-TO-mah): malignant brain tumor composed of immature (-BLAST) neuroglial (supportive nervous tissue) cells.

GLUCOCORTICOID (gloo-ko-KOR-tih-koid): a hormone secreted by the adrenal gland (cortex) to raise blood sugar levels. Examples are cortisone and cortisol.

GLYCOSURIA (gli-ko-SU-re-ah): abnormal condition of sugar in the urine.

GOITER (GOY-ter): enlargement of the thyroid gland.

GOUT (gout): see GOUTY ARTHRITIS.

GOUTY ARTHRITIS (gowti arth-RI-tis): deposits of uric acid crystals in joints and other tissues that cause swelling and inflammation of joints. Also called gout.

GRAVES DISEASE (gravs dih-ZEZ): see HYPERTHYROIDISM.

GROWTH HORMONE (groth HOR-mon): hormone secreted by the pituitary gland to stimulate the growth of bones and the body in general. Also called somatotropin.

GYNECOLOGIST (gi-neh-KOL-o-jist): specialist in the medical and surgical treatment of female disorders.

GYNECOLOGY (gi-neh-KOL-o-je): study of female disorders.

HAIR FOLLICLE (hahr FOL-ih-kl): pouch-like depression in the skin in which a hair develops.

HAIR ROOT (hahr root): part of the hair from which growth occurs.

HDL: see HIGH-DENSITY LIPOPROTEIN.

HEART (hart): hollow, muscular organ in the chest that pumps blood throughout the body.

HEMATEMESIS (he-mah-TEM-eh-sis): vomiting (-EMESIS) of blood (HEMAT/O-).

HEMATOLOGIST (he-mah-TOL-o-jist): specialist in blood and blood disorders.

HEMATOLOGY (he-mah-TOL-o-je): study of the blood.

HEMATOMA (he-mah-TO-mah): mass or collection of blood under the skin. Commonly called a bruise or black-and-blue mark.

HEMATURIA (he-mah-TUR-e-ah): abnormal condition of blood in the urine.

HEMIGASTRECTOMY (heh-me-gas-TREK-to-me): removal of half of the stomach.

HEMIGLOSSECTOMY (hem-e-glos-EK-to-me): removal of half of the tongue.

HEMIPLEGIA (hem-ih-PLE-jah): paralysis of one side of the body.

HEMODIALYSIS (he-mo-di-AL-ih-sis): use of a kidney machine to filter blood to remove waste materials such as urea. Blood leaves the body, enters the machine, and is carried back to the body through a catheter (tube).

HEMOGLOBIN (HE-mo-glo-bin): oxygen-carrying protein found in red blood cells.

HEMOPTYSIS (he-MOP-tih-sis): spitting up (-PTYSIS) of blood (HEM/O-).

HEMORRHAGE (HEM-or-ij): bursting forth of blood.

HEMOTHORAX (he-mo-THOR-aks): collection of blood in the chest (pleural cavity).

HEPATIC (heh-PAT-ik): pertaining to the liver.

HEPATITIS (hep-ah-TI-tis): inflammation of the liver. Viral hepatitis is an acute infectious disease caused by at least three different viruses: hepatitis A, B, and C viruses.

HEPATOMA (hep-ah-TO-mah): tumor (malignant) of the liver; hepatocellular carcinoma.

HEPATOMEGALY (hep-ah-to-MEG-ah-le): enlargement of the liver.

HERNIA (HER-ne-ah): bulge or protrusion of an organ or part of an organ through the wall of the cavity that usually contains it. In an INGUINAL hernia, part of the wall of the abdomen weakens and the intestine bulges out or into the SCROTAL sac (in males).

HIATAL HERNIA (hi-A-tal HER-ne-ah): upward protrusion of the wall of the stomach into the lower part of the esophagus.

HIGH-DENSITY LIPOPROTEIN (hi-DEN-sih-te li-po-PRO-teen): combination of fat and protein in the blood. It carries cholesterol to the liver, which is beneficial.

HIV: see HUMAN IMMUNODEFICIENCY VIRUS.

HODGKIN DISEASE (HOJ-kin di-ZEZ): malignant tumor of lymph nodes.

HORMONE (HOR-mon): chemical made by a gland and sent directly into the bloodstream, not to the outside of the body. ENDOCRINE GLANDS produce hormones.

HUMAN IMMUNODEFICIENCY VIRUS (U-man im-u-no-deh-FISH-en-se VI-rus): virus that infects white blood cells (T cell lymphocytes), causing damage to the patient's immune system. HIV is the cause of AIDS.

HUMERUS (HU-mer-us): upper arm bone.

HYDROCELE (HI-dro-sel): swelling of the SCROTUM caused by a collection of fluid within the outermost covering of the TESTIS.

HYPERGLYCEMIA (hi-per-gli-SE-me-ah): higher than normal levels of sugar in the blood.

HYPERPARATHYROIDISM (hi-per-par-ah-THI-royd-ism): higher than normal level of parathyroid hormone in the blood.

HYPERPLASTIC (hi-per-PLAS-tik): pertaining to excessive growth of normal cells in an organ.

HYPERSECRETION (hi-per-se-KRE-shun): an abnormally high amount of production of a substance.

HYPERTENSION (hi-per-TEN-shun): high blood pressure. *Essential hypertension* has no known cause, but contributing factors are age, obesity, smoking, and heredity. *Secondary hypertension* is a symptom of other disorders such as kidney disease.

HYPERTHYROIDISM (hi-per-THI-royd-izm): excessive activity of the thyroid gland.

HYPERTROPHY (hi-PER-tro-fe): enlargement or overgrowth of an organ or part of the body as a result of an increase in size of individual cells.

HYPODERMIC (hi-po-DER-mik): pertaining to under or below the skin.

HYPOGLYCEMIA (hi-po-gli-SE-me-ah): lower than normal blood sugar levels.

HYPOPHYSEAL (hi-po-FIZ-e-al): pertaining to the pituitary gland.

HYPOPITUITARISM (hi-po-pi-TU-ih-tah-rizm): decrease or stoppage of hormonal secretion by the pituitary gland.

HYPOPLASTIC (hi-po-PLAS-tik): pertaining to underdevelopment of a tissue or organ in the body.

HYPOSECRETION (hi-po-se-KRE-shun): less than normal amount of production of a substance.

HYPOTENSIVE (hi-po-TEN-siv): pertaining to low blood pressure or to a person with abnormally low blood pressure.

HYPOTHYROIDISM (hi-po-THI-royd-izm):   lower than normal activity of the thyroid gland.

HYSTERECTOMY (his-teh-REK-to-me):   excision of the uterus, either through the abdominal wall (abdominal hysterectomy) or through the vagina (vaginal hysterectomy).

HYSTEROSCOPY (his-ter-OS-ko-pe):   visual examination of the uterus using an endoscope inserted through the vagina.

IATROGENIC (i-ah-tro-JEN-ik):   pertaining to a patient's abnormal condition that results unexpectedly from a specific treatment.

ILEOSTOMY (il-e-OS-to-me):   new opening of the ileum (third part of the small intestine) to the outside of the body.

ILEUM (IL-e-um):   third part of the small intestine.

ILIUM (IL-e-um):   side, high portion of the hip bone (pelvis).

INCISION (in-SIZH-un):   cutting into the body or into an organ.

INFARCTION (in-FARK-shun):   area of dead tissue caused by decreased blood flow to that part of the body.

INFECTIOUS DISEASE SPECIALIST (in-FEK-shus dih-ZEZ SPESH-ah-list):   physician who treats disorders caused and spread by microorganisms such as bacteria.

INFILTRATE (IN-fil-trat):   material that accumulates in an organ. The term infiltrate often describes solid material and fluid collection in the lungs.

INFLAMMATORY BOWEL DISEASE (in-FLAM-ah-to-re BOW-el di-ZEZ):   disorder of the small and large intestines marked by bouts of diarrhea, abdominal cramping, and fever. Inflammatory bowel diseases include CROHN DISEASE and ULCERATIVE COLITIS.

INGUINAL (ING-gwi-nal):   pertaining to the groin or the area where the legs meet the body.

INSULIN (IN-su-lin):   hormone produced by the pancreas and released into the bloodstream. Insulin allows sugar to leave the blood and enter body cells.

INTERNAL MEDICINE (in-TER-nal MED-ih-sin):   branch of medicine specializing in the diagnosis of disorders and treatment with drugs.

INTERVERTEBRAL (in-ter-VER-teh-bral):   pertaining to lying between two backbones. A disc (disk) is an intervertebral structure.

INTRA-ABDOMINAL (in-trah-ab-DOM-ih-nal):   pertaining to within the abdomen.

INTRAUTERINE (in-trah-U-ter-in):   pertaining to within the uterus.

INTRAVENOUS (in-trah-VE-nus):   pertaining to within a vein.

INTRAVENOUS PYELOGRAM (in-trah-VEN-nus PI-eh-lo-gram):   x-ray record of the kidney (PYEL/O- means "renal pelvis") after contrast is injected into a vein.

IRIS (I-ris):   colored (pigmented) portion of the eye.

ISCHEMIA (is-KE-me-ah):   deficiency of blood flow to a part of the body, caused by narrowing or obstruction of blood vessels.

JAUNDICE (JAWN-dis):   orange-yellow coloration of the skin and other tissues. A symptom caused by accumulation of BILIRUBIN (pigment) in the blood.

JEJUNUM (jeh-JE-num):   second part of the small intestine.

JOINT (joynt):   space where two or more bones come together (articulate).

KIDNEY (KID-ne):   one of two organs behind the abdomen that produce urine by filtering wastes from the blood.

LAMINECTOMY (lah-men-EK-to-me):   removal of a piece of backbone (lamina) to relieve pressure on nerves from a herniating disc (disk).

LAPAROSCOPE (LAP-ah-ro-skop):   instrument to visually examine the abdomen. An endoscope is inserted through a small incision in the abdominal wall.

LAPAROSCOPIC APPENDECTOMY (lap-ah-ro-SKOP-ik ah-pen-DEK-to-me):   removal of the appendix through a small incision in the abdomen and with the use of a laparoscope.

LAPAROSCOPIC CHOLECYSTECTOMY (lap-ah-ro-SKOP-ik ko-le-sis-TEK-to-me):   removal of the gallbladder through a small incision in the abdomen and with the use of a laparoscopic instrument.

LAPAROSCOPY (lap-ah-ROS-ko-pe):   visual examination of the abdomen. A small incision is made near the navel, and an instrument is inserted to view abdominal organs.

LAPAROTOMY (lap-ah-ROT-o-me):   incision of the abdomen. A surgeon makes a large incision across the abdomen to examine and operate on its organs.

LARGE INTESTINE (larj in-TES-tin):   part of the intestine that receives undigested material from the small intestine and transports it out of the body; the COLON.

LARYNGEAL (lah-rin-JE-al):   pertaining to the larynx (voice box).

LARYNGECTOMY (lah-rin-JEK-to-me):   removal of the larynx (voice box).

LARYNGITIS (lah-rin-JI-tis):   inflammation of the larynx.

LARYNGOSCOPY (lar-in-GOS-ko-pe):   visual examination of the interior of the voice box (larynx) using an endoscope.

LARYNGOTRACHEITIS (lah-ring-o-tra-ke-I-tis):   inflammation of the larynx and the trachea (windpipe).

LARYNX (LAR-inks):   voice box; located at the top of the trachea and containing vocal cords.

LATERAL (LAT-er-al):   pertaining to the side.

LDL: see LOW-DENSITY LIPOPROTEIN.

LEIOMYOMA (li-o-mi-O-mah):   a benign tumor derived from smooth (involuntary) muscle and most often of the uterus (leiomyoma uteri).

LEIOMYOSARCOMA (li-o-mi-o-sar-KO-mah):   a malignant tumor of smooth (involuntary) muscle.

LENS (lenz):   structure behind the pupil of the eye. The lens bends light rays so that they are properly focused on the RETINA at the back of the eye.

LESION (LE-zhun):   any damage to a part of the body, caused by disease or trauma.

LEUKEMIA (lu-KE-me-ah):   excess numbers of malignant white blood cells in the blood and bone marrow.

LEUKOCYTE (LOO-ko-sit):   white blood cell.

LEUKOCYTOSIS (lu-ko-si-TO-sis):   slight increase in the numbers of white blood cells as a response to infection.

LIGAMENT (LIG-ah-ment):   connective tissue that joins bones to other bones.

LIGAMENTOUS (lig-ah-MEN-tus):   pertaining to a LIGAMENT.

LIPOSARCOMA (li-po-sar-KO-mah):   malignant tumor of fatty tissue.

LITHOTRIPSY (lith-o-TRIP-se):   process of crushing a stone in the urinary tract using ultrasonic vibrations.

LIVER (LIV-er):   organ in the right upper quadrant of the abdomen. The liver produces BILE, stores sugar, and produces blood-clotting proteins.

LOBE (lob):   part of an organ, especially of the brain, lungs, or glands.

LOW-DENSITY LIPOPROTEIN (lo-DEN-sih-te li-po-PRO-teen):   combination of lipid (fat) and protein. It has a high CHOLESTEROL content and is associated with forming plaques in arteries.

LOWER GASTROINTESTINAL (GI) SERIES (LOW-er gas-tro-in-TES-tin-al SER-ez):   barium is injected into the anus and rectum and x-rays are taken of the colon (large intestine).

LUMBAR (LUM-bar):   pertaining to the loins; part of the back and sides between the chest and the hip.

LUMBAR REGION (LUM-bar RE-jin):   pertaining to the backbones that lie between the thoracic (chest) and sacral (lower back) vertebrae.

LUMBAR VERTEBRA (LUM-bar VER-teh-brah):   a backbone in the region between the chest and lower back.

LUNG (lung):   one of two paired organs in the chest through which oxygen enters and carbon dioxide leaves the body.

LUNG CAPILLARIES (lung KAP-ih-lar-ez):   tiny blood vessels surrounding lung tissue and through which gases pass into and out of the bloodstream.

LUPUS ERYTHEMATOSUS: see SYSTEMIC LUPUS ERYTHEMATOSUS.

LYMPH (limf):   clear fluid that is found in lymph vessels and produced from fluid surrounding cells. Lymph contains white blood cells (lymphocytes) that fight disease.

LYMPHADENECTOMY (limf-ah-deh-NEK-to-me):   removal of LYMPH NODES.

LYMPHADENOPATHY (lim-fad-eh-NOP-ah-the):   disease of lymph nodes (glands).

LYMPHANGIOGRAM (LIMFAN-je-o-gram):   x-ray record of lymph vessels after contrast is injected into soft tissue of the foot.

LYMPHANGIOGRAPHY (limfan-je-OG-ra-fe):   x-ray examination of lymph vessels and nodes after the injection of contrast medium into the soft tissue of the foot.

LYMPHATIC SYSTEM (lim-FAT-ik SIS-tem):   group of organs (lymph vessels, lymph nodes, spleen, thymus) composed of lymphatic tissue that produce lymphocytes to defend the body against foreign organisms.

LYMPHATIC VESSELS (lim-FAT-ik VES-elz):   tubes that carry lymph from tissues to the bloodstream (into a vein in the neck region); lymph vessels.

LYMPHEDEMA (limf-ah-DE-mah):   accumulation of fluid in tissue spaces, causing swelling. Lymphedema is caused by the obstruction of lymph nodes or vessels.

LYMPH NODE (limf nod):   stationary collection of lymph cells, found all over the body. Lymph nodes are sometimes called lymph glands.

LYMPHOCYTE (LIMF-o-site):   white blood cell that is found within lymph and lymph nodes. T cells and B cells are types of lymphocytes.

LYMPHOID (LIM-foid):   resembling or pertaining to lymph tissue.

LYMPHOMA (lim-FO-mah):   malignant tumor of lymphatic tissue. Previously called lymphosarcoma.

MAGNETIC RESONANCE IMAGING (mag-NET-ik REZ-o-nans IM-aj-ing): image of the body using magnetic and radio waves. Organs are seen in three planes: frontal (front to back), sagittal (side to side), and transverse (cross-section). Called *MRI*.

MALE REPRODUCTIVE SYSTEM (mal re-pro-DUK-tiv SIS-tem): organs that produce sperm cells and male hormones.

MALIGNANT (mah-LIG-nant): tending to become progressively worse. The term malignant describes cancerous tumors that invade and spread to distant organs.

MAMMARY (MAM-er-e): pertaining to the breast.

MAMMOGRAM (MAM-o-gram): x-ray record of the breast.

MAMMOGRAPHY (mam-MOG-ra-fe): process of making an x-ray recording of the breast.

MAMMOPLASTY (MAM-o-plas-te): surgical repair (reconstruction) of the breast.

MASTECTOMY (mas-TEK-to-me): removal (excision) of the breast.

MASTITIS (mas-TI-tis): inflammation of the breast.

MEDIASTINAL (me-de-ah-STI-nal): pertaining to the MEDIASTINUM.

MEDIASTINOSCOPY (me-de-ah-sti-NOS-ko-pe): visual examination of the mediastinum using an endoscope.

MEDIASTINUM (me-de-ah-STI-num): space between the lungs in the chest. The mediastinum contains the heart, large blood vessels, trachea, esophagus, thymus gland, and lymph nodes.

MEDULLA OBLONGATA (meh-DUL-ah ob-lon-GA-tah): lower part of the brain near the spinal cord. The medulla oblongata controls breathing and heartbeat.

MEDULLARY (MEH-DU-lar-e): pertaining to the inner, or soft, part of an organ.

MELANOMA (meh-lah-NO-mah): malignant tumor arising from pigmented cells (melanocytes) in the skin. A melanoma usually develops from a NEVUS (mole).

MENINGES (meh-NIN-jes): membranes surrounding the brain and spinal cord.

MENINGITIS (men-in-JI-tis): inflammation of the meninges (membranes around the brain and spinal cord).

MENORRHAGIA (men-or-RA-jah): excessive bleeding from the uterus during the time of MENSTRUATION.

MENORRHEA (men-o-RE-ah): normal discharge of blood and tissue from the uterine lining during MENSTRUATION.

MENSES (MEN-sez): menstruation; menstrual period.

MENSTRUATION (men-stru-A-shun): breakdown of the lining of the uterus that occurs every four weeks during the active reproductive period of a female.

MESOTHELIOMA (mes-o-the-le-O-mah): malignant tumor of the lining tissue (mesothelium) of the pleura. A mesothelioma is associated with exposure to asbestos.

METACARPALS (met-ah-KAR-palz): bones of the hand between the wrist bones (carpals) and the finger bones (phalanges).

METASTASIS (meh-TAS-tah-sis): spread of a cancerous tumor to a distant organ or location. Metastasis literally means "change" (META-) of "place" (-STASIS).

METATARSALS (meh-tah-TAR-sels): foot bones.

MIGRAINE (MI-gran): attack of headache, usually on one side of the head, caused by changes in blood vessel size and accompanied by nausea, vomiting, and sensitivity to light (photophobia). Migraine is a term from the French word *migraine,* meaning "severe head pain."

MINIMALLY INVASIVE SURGERY (MIN-ih-mal-le in-VA-siv SUR-jer-e): removal and repair of organs and tissues using small incisions for an endoscope (laparoscope) and instruments. Examples are laparoscopic cholecystectomy (gallbladder removal), laparoscopic appendectomy (appendix removal), laparoscopic herniorrhaphy (repair of a hernia), and laparoscopic colectomy (removal of a portion of the colon).

MONOCYTE (MON-o-sit): white blood cell with one large nucleus.

MONONUCLEOSIS (mon-o-nu-kle-O-sis): an acute infectious disease with excess MONOCYTES in the blood. Mononucleosis is caused by the Epstein-Barr virus and is transmitted by direct oral (mouth) contact.

MOUTH (mowth): the opening that forms the beginning of the digestive system.

MRI: see MAGNETIC RESONANCE IMAGING.

MULTIPLE MYELOMA (MUL-tih-pul mi-eh-LO-mah): malignant tumor of the bone marrow.

MULTIPLE SCLEROSIS (MUL-tih-pul skeh-RO-sis): chronic neurological disease in which there are patches of loss of MYELIN SHEATH (covering neurons) throughout the brain and spinal cord. Weakness, abnormal sensations, incoordination, and speech and visual disturbances are symptoms.

MUSCLE (MUS-el): connective tissue that contracts to make movement possible.

MUSCULAR (MUS-ku-lar): pertaining to muscles.

MUSCULAR DYSTROPHY (MUS-ku-lar DIS-tro-fe): group of degenerative muscle diseases that cause crippling because muscles are gradually weakened and eventually ATROPHY (shrink).

MUSCULOSKELETAL SYSTEM (mus-ku-lo-SKEL-e-tal SIS-tem): organs that support the body and allow it to move, including the muscles, bones, joints, and connective tissues.

MYALGIA (mi-AL-jah): pain in a muscle or muscles.

MYELIN SHEATH (MI-eh-lin sheth): fatty covering around part (axon) of some nerve fibers. The myelin sheath insulates and speeds the conduction of nerve impulses.

MYELODYSPLASIA (mi-eh-lo-dis-PLA-ze-ah): abnormal development of bone marrow, a premalignant condition leading to leukemia.

MYELOGRAM (MI-eh-lo-gram): x-ray record of the spinal cord after contrast is injected within the membranes surrounding the spinal cord in the lumbar area of the back.

MYELOGRAPHY (mi-eh-LOG-rah-fe): process of recording the spinal cord after injection of contrast material.

MYELOMA (mi-eh-LO-mah): malignant tumor originating in the bone marrow (MYEL/O-). Also called MULTIPLE MYELOMA.

MYOCARDIAL (mi-o-KAR-de-al): pertaining to the muscle of the heart.

MYOCARDIAL INFARCTION (mi-o-KAR-de-al in-FARK-shun): area of dead tissue in heart muscle; also known as a heart attack or an MI.

MYOCARDIAL ISCHEMIA (mi-o-KAR-de-al is-KE-me-ah): decrease in the blood supply to the heart muscle.

MYOMA (mi-O-mah): tumor (benign) of muscle.

MYOMECTOMY (mi-o-MEK-to-me): removal of a benign muscle tumor (fibroid).

MYOSARCOMA (mi-o-sar-KO-mah):   tumor (malignant) of muscle. SARC- means "flesh," indicating that the tumor is of connective or "fleshy" tissue origin.

MYOSITIS (mi-o-SI-tis):   inflammation of a muscle.

MYRINGOTOMY (mir-in-GOT-o-me):   incision of the eardrum.

NASAL (NA-zel):   pertaining to the nose.

NAUSEA (NAW-se-ah):   unpleasant sensation in the upper abdomen, often leading to vomiting. The term comes from the Greek *nausia,* meaning "sea sickness."

NECROSIS (neh-KRO-sis):   death of cells.

NECROTIC (neh-KRO-tik):   pertaining to death of cells.

NEONATAL (ne-o-NA-tal):   pertaining to new birth; the first four weeks after birth.

NEOPLASM (NE-o-plazm):   any new growth of tissue; a tumor.

NEOPLASTIC (ne-o-PLAS-tik):   pertaining to a new growth, or NEOPLASM.

NEPHRECTOMY (neh-FREK-to-me):   removal (excision) of a kidney.

NEPHRITIS (neh-FRI-tis):   inflammation of kidneys.

NEPHROLITHIASIS (neh-fro-lih-THI-ah-sis):   condition of kidney stones.

NEPHROLOGIST (neh-FROL-o-jist):   specialist in the diagnosis and treatment of kidney diseases.

NEPHROLOGY (neh-FROL-o-je):   study of the kidney and its diseases.

NEPHROPATHY (neh-FROP-ah-the):   disease of the kidney.

NEPHROSIS (neh-FRO-sis):   abnormal condition of the kidney. Nephrosis is often associated with a deterioration of the kidney tubules.

NEPHROSTOMY (neh-FROS-to-me):   opening from the kidney to the outside of the body.

NERVOUS SYSTEM (NER-vus SIS-tem):   organs (brain, spinal cord, and nerves) that transmit electrical messages throughout the body.

NEURAL (NU-ral):   pertaining to nerves.

NEURALGIA (nu-RAL-jah):   nerve pain.

NEURITIS (nu-RI-tis):   inflammation of a nerve.

NEUROGLIAL CELLS (nu-ro-GLE-al selz):   supporting structure of nervous tissue in the central nervous system, such as the brain. Examples are astrocytes, microglial, and oligodendroglial cells. These cells are often the source of brain tumors.

NEUROLOGIST (nu-ROL-o-jist):   specialist in the diagnosis and treatment of nervous disorders.

NEUROLOGY (nu-ROL-o-je):   study of the nervous system and nerve disorders.

NEUROPATHY (nu-ROP-ah-the):   disease of nervous tissue.

NEUROSURGEON (nu-ro-SUR-jin):   physician who operates on the organs of the nervous system (brain, spinal cord, and nerves).

NEUROTOMY (nu-ROT-o-me):   incision of a nerve.

NEVUS (NE-vus):   pigmented lesion on the skin; a mole.

NOCTURIA (nok-TU-re-ah):   excessive urination at night.

NOSE (noz):   structure that is the organ of smell and permits air to enter and leave the body.

NOSOCOMIAL (nos-o-KO-me-al):   pertaining to or originating in a hospital. A nosocomial infection is acquired during hospitalization.

OBSTETRIC (ob-STEH-TRIK):   pertaining to pregnancy, labor, and delivery of a baby.

OBSTETRICIAN (ob-steh-TRISH-un):   specialist in the delivery of a baby and care of the mother during pregnancy and labor.

OBSTETRICS (ob-STET-riks):   practice or branch of medicine concerned with the management of women during pregnancy, childbirth, and the period just after delivery of the infant.

OCULAR (OK-u-lar):   pertaining to the eye.

ONCOGENIC (ong-ko-JEN-ik):   pertaining to producing (-GEN) tumors.

ONCOLOGIST (ong-KOL-o-jist):   physician specializing in the study and treatment of tumors.

ONCOLOGY (ong-KOL-o-je):   study of tumors.

OOPHORECTOMY (o-of-o-REK-to-me or oo-fo-REK-to-me):   removal of an ovary or ovaries.

OOPHORITIS (o-of-o-RI-tis or oo-pho-RI-tis):   inflammation of an ovary.

OPHTHALMOLOGIST (of-thal-MOL-o-jist):   specialist in the study of the eye and the treatment of eye disorders.

OPHTHALMOLOGY (of-thal-MOL-o-je):   study of the eye; the diagnosis and treatment of eye disorders.

OPHTHALMOSCOPE (of-THAL-mo-scop):   instrument used to visually examine the eye.

OPTIC NERVE (OP-tik nerv):   nerve in the back of the eye that transmits light waves to the brain.

OPTICIAN (op-TISH-an):   non-medical specialist trained to provide eyeglasses by filling prescriptions.

OPTOMETRIST (op-TOM-eh-trist):   non-medical specialist trained to examine and test eyes and prescribe corrective lenses.

ORAL (OR-al):   pertaining to the mouth.

ORCHIDECTOMY (or-kih-DEK-to-me):   removal (excision) of a testicle or testicles.

ORCHIECTOMY (or-ke-EK-to-me):   removal (excision) of a testicle or testicles.

ORCHIOPEXY (or-ke-o-PEK-se):   surgical fixation of the testicle (testis) into its proper location within the scrotum. This surgery corrects CRYPTORCHISM.

ORCHITIS (or-KI-tis):   inflammation of a testicle.

ORGAN (OR-gan):   independent part of the body composed of different tissues working together to do a specific job.

ORTHOPEDIST (or-tho-PE-dist):   specialist in the surgical correction of musculoskeletal disorders. This physician was originally concerned with straightening (ORTH/O-) bones in the legs of deformed children (PED/O-).

OSTEITIS (os-te-I-tis):   inflammation of a bone.

OSTEOARTHRITIS (os-te-o-ar-THRI-tis):   inflammation of bones and joints. Osteoarthritis is a disease of older people and is marked by stiffness, pain, and degeneration of joints.

OSTEOGENIC SARCOMA (os-te-o-JEN-ik sar-KO-mah):   malignant (cancerous) tumor of bone (-GENIC means "produced in").

OSTEOMA (os-te-O-mah):   tumor (benign) of bone.

OSTEOMYELITIS (os-te-o-mi-eh-LI-tis): inflammation of bone and bone marrow. Osteomyelitis is caused by a bacterial infection.

OSTEOPOROSIS (os-te-o-po-RO-sis): decrease in bone mass with formation of pores or spaces in normally mineralized bone tissue.

OSTEOTOMY (os-te-OT-o-me): incision of a bone.

OTALGIA (o-TAL-jah): pain in an ear.

OTITIS (o-TI-tis): inflammation of an ear.

OTOLARYNGOLOGIST (o-to-lah-rin-GOL-o-jist): specialist in the treatment of diseases of the ear, nose, and throat.

OVARIAN (o-VAR-e-an): pertaining to an OVARY or ovaries.

OVARIAN CANCER (o-VAR-e-an KAN-ser): malignant condition of the ovaries.

OVARIAN CYST (o-VAR-e-an sist): sac containing fluid or semi-solid material in or on the ovary.

OVARY (O-vah-re): one of two organs in the female abdomen that produces egg cells and female hormones.

OVUM (O-vum): egg cell (pl. ova [o-VAH]).

OXYGEN (OK-si-jen): colorless, odorless gas that is essential to sustaining life.

PANCREAS (PAN-kre-us): gland that produces digestive juices (exocrine function) and the hormone INSULIN (endocrine function).

PANCREATECTOMY (pan-kre-ah-TEK-to-me): removal of the pancreas.

PANCREATITIS (pan-kre-ah-TI-tis): inflammation of the pancreas.

PARALYSIS (pah-RAL-ih-sis): loss or impairment of movement in a part of the body.

PARAPLEGIA (par-ah-PLE-jah): impairment or loss of movement in the lower part of the body, primarily the legs and in some cases bowel and bladder function.

PARATHYROID GLANDS (par-ah-THI-royd glanz): four endocrine glands behind the thyroid gland. These glands are concerned with maintaining the proper levels of calcium in the blood and bones.

PARATHYROID HORMONE (par-ah-THI-roid HOR-mon): hormone secreted by the parathyroid glands to maintain a constant concentration of calcium in the blood and bones. Also called PTH.

PATELLA (pah-TEL-ah): knee cap.

PATHOLOGIST (pah-THOL-o-jist): specialist in the study of disease using microscopic examination of tissues and cells and autopsy examination.

PATHOLOGY (pah-THOL-o-je): study of disease.

PEDIATRIC (pe-de-AT-rik): pertaining to treatment of a child.

PEDIATRICIAN (pe-de-ah-TRISH-un): specialist in the treatment of childhood diseases.

PEDIATRICS (pe-de-AT-riks): branch of medicine specializing in the treatment of children.

PELVIC (PEL-vik): pertaining to the hip bone (pelvis) or the region of the hip.

PELVIC CAVITY (PEL-vik KAV-ih-te): space contained within the hip bone (front and sides) and the lower part of the backbone (sacrum and coccyx).

PELVIC INFLAMMATORY DISEASE (PEL-vik in-FLAM-ah-to-re di-ZEZ): inflammation in the pelvic region; usually, inflammation of the fallopian tubes.

PELVIS (PEL-vis): hip bone. The pelvis is composed of the ilium (upper portion), ischium (lower portion), and pubis (front portion).

PENICILLIN (pen-in-SIL-in): substance, derived from certain molds, that can destroy bacteria; an ANTIBIOTIC.

PENIS (PE-nis): external male organ containing the urethra, through which both urine and semen (sperm cells and fluid) leave the body.

PEPTIC ULCER (PEP-tik UL-ser): sore (lesion) of the mucous membrane lining the first part of the small intestine (duodenum) or lining the stomach.

PERCUTANEOUS (per-ku-TAN-e-us): pertaining to through the skin.

PERCUTANEOUS TRANSHEPATIC CHOLANGIOGRAPHY (per-ku-TAN-e-us trans-heh-PAT-ik kol-an-je-OG-rah-fe): bile vessels are imaged after injection of contrast material through the skin into the liver.

PERIANAL (per-e-A-nal): pertaining to surrounding the ANUS.

PERIOSTEUM (per-e-OS-te-um): membrane that surrounds bone.

PERITONEAL (per-ih-to-NE-al): pertaining to the PERITONEUM.

PERITONEAL DIALYSIS (per-ih-to-NE-al di-AL-ih-sis): process of removing wastes from the blood by introducing a special fluid into the abdomen. The wastes pass into the fluid from the bloodstream, and then the fluid is drained from the body.

PERITONEOSCOPY (per-ih-to-ne-OS-ko-pe): visual examination of the peritoneal cavity using an endoscope. See LAPAROSCOPY.

PERITONEUM (per-ih-to-NE-um): membrane that surrounds the abdomen and holds the abdominal organs in place.

PERITONITIS (per-ih-to-NI-tis): inflammation of the peritoneum.

PHALANGES (fah-LAN-jez): finger and toe bones.

PHARYNGEAL (fah-rin-JE-al): pertaining to the pharynx (throat).

PHARYNGITIS (fah-rin-JI-tis): inflammation of the pharynx (throat).

PHARYNX (FAR-inks): organ behind the mouth that receives swallowed food and delivers it into the esophagus. The pharynx (throat) also receives air from the nose and passes it to the trachea (windpipe).

PHENOTHIAZINE (fe-no-THI-ah-zen): substance whose derivatives are used as tranquilizers and antipsychotic agents to treat mental illness.

PHLEBITIS (fleh-BI-tis): inflammation of a vein.

PHLEBOGRAPHY (fle-BOG-ra-fe): x-ray examination of veins after injecting contrast material.

PHLEBOTOMY (fleh-BOT-o-me): incision of a vein.

PHRENIC (FREH-nik): pertaining to the DIAPHRAGM.

PHYSICAL MEDICINE AND REHABILITATION (FIZ-e-kal MED-i-sin and re-ha-bil-i-TA-shun): field of medicine that specializes in restoring the function of the body after illness.

PINEAL GLAND (pi-NE-al gland): small endocrine gland within the brain that secretes the hormone melatonin, whose exact function is unclear. In lower animals the pineal gland is a receptor for light.

PITUITARY GLAND (pih-TU-ih-tar-e gland): organ at the base of the brain that secretes hormones. These hormones enter the blood to regulate other organs and other endocrine glands.

PLATELET (PLAT-let): cell in the blood that aids clotting; a thrombocyte.

PLEURA (PLOO-rah): double membrane that surrounds the lungs.

PLEURAL CAVITY (PLOO-ral KA-vih-te): space between the pleura surrounding the lungs.

PLEURAL EFFUSION (PLOO-ral e-FU-zhun): collection of fluid between the double membrane surrounding the lungs.

PLEURISY (PLOO-ih-se): inflammation of the PLEURA.

PLEURITIS (ploo-RI-tis): inflammation of the PLEURA.

PNEUMOCONIOSIS (noo-mo-ko-ne-O-sis): group of lung diseases resulting from inhalation of particles of dust such as coal, with permanent deposition of such particles in the lung.

PNEUMONECTOMY (noo-mo-NEK-to-me): removal of a lung.

PNEUMONIA (noo-MO-ne-ah): abnormal condition of the lungs marked by inflammation and collection of material within the air sacs of the lungs.

PNEUMONITIS (noo-mo-NI-tis): inflammation of a lung or lungs.

PNEUMOTHORAX (noo-mo-THO-raks): abnormal accumulation of air in the space between the pleura.

POLYCYTHEMIA (pol-e-si-THE-me-ah): increase in red blood cells. One form of polycythemia is polycythemia vera, in which the bone marrow produces an excess of erythrocytes.

POLYDIPSIA (pol-e-DIP-se-ah): excessive thirst.

POLYNEUROPATHY (pol-e-nu-ROP-ah-the): disease of many nerves.

POLYP (POL-ip): a growth or mass (benign) protruding from a mucous membrane, and hemoglobin level is elevated.

POLYURIA (pol-e-UR-e-ah): excessive urination.

POST MORTEM (post MOR-tem): after death.

POST PARTUM (post PAR-tum): after birth.

POSTERIOR (pos-TER-e-or): located in the back portion of a structure or of the body.

PRECANCEROUS (pre-KAN-ser-us): pertaining to a condition that may come before a cancer; a condition that tends to become malignant.

PRENATAL (pre-NA-tal): pertaining to before birth.

PROCTOLOGIST (prok-TOL-o-jist): physician who specializes in the study of the anus and rectum.

PROCTOSCOPY (prok-TOS-ko-pe): inspection of the anus and rectum with a proctoscope (ENDOSCOPE). Proctoscopy is often performed before rectal surgery.

PROCTOSIGMOIDOSCOPY (prok-to-sig-moyd-OS-ko-pe): visual examination of the anus, rectum, and sigmoid colon using an endoscope.

PROGESTERONE (pro-JES-teh-rone): hormone secreted by the ovaries to prepare to maintain the uterine lining during pregnancy.

PROGNOSIS (prog-NO-sis): forecast as to the probable outcome of an illness or treatment. Prognosis literally means "before" (PRO-) "knowledge" (-GNOSIS).

PROLAPSE (pro-LAPS): falling down or drooping of a part of the body Prolapse literally means "sliding" (-LAPSE) "forward" (PRO-).

PROSTATE GLAND (PROS-tat gland): male gland that surrounds the base of the urinary bladder. It produces fluid that leaves the body with sperm cells.

PROSTATECTOMY (pros-tah-TEK-to-me): removal of the prostate gland.

PROSTATIC (pros-TAH-tik):   pertaining to the prostate gland.

PROSTATIC CARCINOMA (pros-TAH-tik kar-si-NO-mah):   malignant tumor arising from the PROSTATE GLAND.

PROSTATIC HYPERPLASIA (pros-TAH-tik hi-per-PLA-zhah):   abnormal increase in growth (benign) of the prostate gland.

PROSTHESIS (pros-THE-sis):   artificial substitute for a missing part of the body. Prosthesis literally means "to place" (-THESIS) "before" (PROS-).

PROTEINURIA (pro-en-U-re-ah):   abnormal condition of protein in the urine (albuminuria).

PSYCHIATRIST (si-KI-ah-trist):   specialist in the treatment of the mind and mental disorders.

PSYCHIATRY (si-KI-ah-tre):   treatment (IATR/O-) of disorders of the mind (PSYCH/O-).

PSYCHOLOGY (si-KOL-o-je):   study of the mind, especially in relation to human behavior.

PSYCHOSIS (si-KO-sis):   abnormal condition of the mind; a serious mental disorder that involves loss of normal perception of reality (pl. psychoses [si-KO-sez]).

PULMONARY (PUL-mo-ner-e):   pertaining to the lungs.

PULMONARY CIRCULATION (PUL-mo-ner-e ser-ku-LA-shun):   passage of blood from the heart to the lungs and back to the heart.

PULMONARY EDEMA (PUL-mo-ner-e eh-DE-mah):   abnormal collection of fluid in the lung (within the air sacs of the lung).

PULMONARY EMBOLISM (PUL-mo-ner-e EM-bo-lizm):   blockage of blood vessels by foreign matter (clot, tumor, fat, or air). The embolus frequently arises from the deep veins of the leg.

PULMONARY SPECIALIST (PUL-mo-ner-e SPESH-ah-list):   physician trained to treat lung disorders.

PUPIL (PU-pil):   black center of the eye through which light enters.

PYELITIS (pi-eh-LI-tis):   inflammation of the renal pelvis (central section of the kidney).

PYELOGRAM (PI-lo-gram):   record of the renal pelvis after injection of contrast.

QUADRIPLEGIA (kwod-ri-PLE-jah):   paralysis of all four extremities and usually the trunk of the body caused by injury to the spinal cord in the cervical region of the spine.

RADIATION ONCOLOGIST (ra-de-A-shun ong-KOL-o-jist):   physician trained in the treatment of disease (cancer) using high-energy x-rays or other particles.

RADIOLOGIST (ra-de-OL-o-jist):   physician trained in the use of x-rays (including ultrasound and magnetic resonance imaging techniques) to diagnose illness.

RADIOLOGY (ra-de-OL-o-je):   science of using x-rays in the diagnosis of disease.

RADIOTHERAPY (ra-de-o-THER-ah-pe):   treatment of disease (cancer) using high-energy particles such as x-rays and protons.

RADIUS (RA-de-us):   one of two lower arm bones. The radius is located on the thumb side of the hand.

RECTAL RESECTION (REK-tal re-SEK-shun):   excision (resection) of the RECTUM.

RECTOCELE (REK-to-sel):   hernia (protrusion) of the rectum into the vagina.

RECTUM (REK-tum):   end of the colon. The rectum delivers wastes (feces) to the anus for elimination.

RELAPSE (re-LAPS):   return of disease after its apparent termination.

REMISSION (re-MISH-un):   lessening of symptoms of a disease.

RENAL (RE-nal):   pertaining to the kidney.

RENAL FAILURE (RE-nal FAL-ur):   kidneys no longer function.

RENAL PELVIS (RE-nal PEL-vis):   central section of the kidney, where urine collects.

REPRODUCTIVE (re-pro-DUK-tiv):   pertaining to the process by which living things produce offspring.

RESEARCH (RE-surch):   laboratory investigation of a medical problem.

RESECTION (re-SEK-shun):   removal of an organ or a structure.

RESIDENCY TRAINING (RES-i-den-se TRAY-ning):   period of hospital work involving the care of patients after the completion of four years of medical school.

RESPIRATORY SYSTEM (RES-pir-ah-tor-e SIS-tem):   organs that control breathing, allowing air to enter and leave the body.

RETINA (RET-ih-nah):   layer of sensitive cells at the back of the eye. Light is focused on the retina and then is transmitted to the optic nerve, which leads to the brain.

RETINOPATHY (reh-tih-NOP-ah-the):   disease of the RETINA.

RETROGASTRIC (reh-tro-GAS-trik):   pertaining to behind the stomach.

RETROPERITONEAL (reh-tro-per-ih-to-NE-al):   pertaining to behind the PERITONEUM.

RHABDOMYOSARCOMA (rab-do-mi-o-sar-KO-mah):   a malignant tumor of muscle cells (skeletal, voluntary muscle) that occurs most frequently in the head and neck, extremities, body wall, and area behind the abdomen.

RHEUMATOID ARTHRITIS (ROO-mah-toyd arth-RI-tis):   chronic inflammatory disease of the joints and connective tissue that leads to deformed joints.

RHEUMATOLOGIST (roo-mah-TOL-o-jist):   specialist in the treatment of diseases of connective tissues, especially the joints. RHEUMAT/O- comes from the Greek *rheuma,* meaning "that which flows, as a stream or a river." Inflammatory disorders of joints are often marked by a collection of fluid in joint spaces.

RHEUMATOLOGY (roo-mah-TOL-o-je):   branch of medicine dealing with inflammation, degeneration, or chemical changes in connective tissues, such as joints and muscles. Pain, stiffness, or limitation of motion are often characteristics of rheumatologic disorders.

RHINITIS (ri-NI-tis):   inflammation of the nose.

RHINOPLASTY (RI-no-plas-te):   surgical repair of the nose.

RHINORRHEA (ri-no-RE-ah):   discharge from the nose.

RHINOTOMY (ri-NOT-o-me):   incision of the nose.

RIB (rib):   one of twelve paired bones surrounding the chest. Seven ribs (true ribs) attach directly to the breastbone, three (false ribs) attach to the seventh rib, and two (floating ribs) are not attached at all.

SACRAL (SA-kral):   pertaining to the SACRUM.

SACRAL REGION (SA-kral RE-jin):   five fused bones in the lower back, below the lumbar bones and wedged between two parts of the hip (ilium).

SACRUM (SA-krum):   triangular bone in the lower back, below the lumbar bones and formed by five fused bones.

SAGITTAL PLANE (SAJ-ih-tal plan):   an imaginary line that divides an organ or the body into right and left portions.

SAGITTAL SECTION (SAJ-ih-tal SEK-shun):   cut (section) through the body dividing it into a right and left portion.

SALPINGECTOMY (sal-pin-JEK-to-me):   removal of a fallopian (uterine) tube.

SALPINGITIS (sal-pin-JI-tis):   inflammation of a fallopian (uterine) tube.

SARCOIDOSIS (sahr-koi-DO-sis):   chronic, progressive disorder of cells in connective tissue, spleen, liver, bone marrow, lungs, and lymph nodes. Small collections of cells (granulomas) form in affected organs and tissues.

SARCOMA (sar-KO-mah):   cancerous (malignant) tumor of connective tissue, such as bone, muscle, fat, or cartilage.

SCAPULA (SKAP-u-lah):   shoulder bone.

SCLERA (SKLE-rah):   white, outer coat of the eyeball.

SCROTAL (SKRO-tal):   pertaining to the scrotum.

SCROTUM (SKRO-tum):   sac on the outside of the body that contains the testes.

SEBACEOUS GLAND (seh-BA-shus gland):   oil-producing (sebum-producing) gland in the skin.

SECTION (SEK-shun):   an act of cutting; a segment or subdivision of an organ.

SEIZURE (SE-zhur):   convulsion (involuntary contraction of muscles) or attack of EPILEPSY. A seizure can also indicate a sudden attack or recurrence of a disease.

SELLA TURCICA (SEL-ah TUR-sih-ka):   cup-like depression at the base of the skull that holds the pituitary gland.

SEMEN (SE-men):   fluid composed of sperm cells and secretions from the prostate gland and other male exocrine glands.

SEMINOMA (sem-ih-NO-mah):   malignant tumor of the testis.

SENSE ORGANS (sens OR-ganz):   parts of the body that receive messages from the environment and relay them to the brain so that we see, hear, and feel sensations. Examples of sense organs are the eye, the ear, and the skin.

SEPTIC (SEP-tik):   pertaining to infection.

SEPTICEMIA (sep-tih-SE-me-ah):   infection in the blood. Septicemia is commonly called blood poisoning and is associated with the presence of bacteria or their poisons in the blood.

SHOCK (shok):   group of symptoms (pale skin, rapid pulse, shallow breathing) that indicate poor oxygen supply to tissue and insufficient return of blood to the heart.

SIGMOID COLON (SIG-moyd KO-len):   S-shaped lower portion of the colon.

SIGMOIDOSCOPY (sig-moyd-OS-ko-pe):   visual examination of the sigmoid colon using an endoscope inserted through the anus and rectum.

SKIN (skin):   outer covering that protects the body.

SKULL (skul):   bone that surrounds the brain and other organs in the head.

SMALL INTESTINE (smal in-TES-tin):   organ that receives food from the stomach. The small intestine is divided into three sections: duodenum, jejunum, and ileum.

SONOGRAM (SON-o-gram):   record of sound waves after they bounce off organs in the body; an ULTRASOUND or echogram.

SPERMATOZOON (sper-mah-to-ZO-on): sperm cell (pl. spermatozoa [sper-mah-to-ZO-ah]).

SPINAL (SPI-nal): pertaining to the spine (backbone).

SPINAL CAVITY (SPI-nal KAV-ih-te): space in the back that contains the spinal cord and is surrounded by the backbones.

SPINAL COLUMN (SPI-nal KOL-um): backbones; vertebrae.

SPINAL CORD (SPI-nal kord): bundle of nerves that extends from the brain down the back. The spinal cord carries electrical messages to and from the spinal cord.

SPINAL NERVES (SPI-nal nervz): nerves that transmit messages to and from the spinal cord.

SPLEEN (splen): organ in the left upper quadrant of the abdomen. The spleen stores blood cells and destroys red blood cells while producing white blood cells called LYMPHOCYTES.

SPLENECTOMY (splen-EK-to-me): removal of the spleen.

SPLENOMEGALY (splehn-o-MEG-ah-le): enlargement of the spleen.

SPONDYLITIS (spon-dih-LI-tis): chronic, serious inflammatory disorder of backbones involving erosion and collapse of vertebrae. See ANKYLOSING SPONDYLITIS.

SPONDYLOSIS (spon-dih-LO-sis): abnormal condition of a vertebra or vertebrae.

SPUTUM (SPU-tum): material expelled from the lungs and expelled through the mouth.

STERNUM (STER-num): breast bone.

STOMACH (STUM-ak): organ that receives food from the esophagus and sends it to the small intestine. Enzymes in the stomach break down food particles during digestion.

STOMATITIS (sto-mah-TI-tis): inflammation of the mouth.

STROKE (strok): Trauma to or blockage of blood vessels within the brain, leading to a reduction in the blood supply to brain tissue. This causes nerve cells in the brain to die and results in loss of function to the part of the body controlled by those nerve cells.

SUBCOSTAL (sub-KOS-tal): pertaining to below the ribs.

SUBCUTANEOUS TISSUE (sub-ku-TA-ne-us TIS-u): lower layer of the skin composed of fatty tissue.

SUBDURAL HEMATOMA (sub-DUR-al he-mah-TO-mah): collection of blood under the dura mater (outermost layer of the membranes surrounding the brain).

SUBGASTRIC (sub-GAS-trik): pertaining to below the stomach.

SUBHEPATIC (sub-heh-PAT-ik): pertaining to under the liver.

SUBSCAPULAR (sub-SKAP-u-lar): pertaining to under the shoulder bone.

SUBTOTAL (sub-TO-tal): less than total; just under the total amount.

SUPRARENAL GLANDS (soo-prah-RE-nal glanz): two endocrine glands, each located above a kidney. Also called adrenal glands.

SURGERY (SUR-jer-e): branch of medicine that treats disease by manual (hand) or operative methods.

SWEAT GLAND (sweht gland): organ in the skin that produces a watery substance containing salts.

SYNCOPE (SING-kah-pe): fainting; sudden loss of consciousness.

SYNDROME (SIN-drom): set of symptoms and signs of disease that occur together to indicate a disease condition.

SYSTEM (SIS-tem): group of organs working together to do a job in the body. For example, the digestive system includes the mouth, throat, stomach, and intestines, all of which help to bring food into the body, break it down, and deliver it to the bloodstream.

SYSTEMIC CIRCULATION (sis-TEM-ik ser-ku-LA-shun): passage of blood from the heart to the tissues of the body and back to the heart.

SYSTEMIC LUPUS ERYTHEMATOSUS (sis-TEM-ik LOO-pus er-ih-the-mah-TO-SUS): chronic inflammatory disease affecting many systems of the body (joints, skin, kidneys, and nerves). A red (erythematous) rash over the nose and cheeks is characteristic.

TACHYCARDIA (tak-eh-KAR-de-ah): condition of fast, rapid heartbeat.

TACHYPNEA (tak-ip-NE-ah): condition of rapid breathing.

TENDINITIS (ten-dih-NI-tis): inflammation of a tendon.

TENDON (TEN-don): connective tissue that joins muscles to bones.

TENORRHAPHY (ten-OR-ah-fe): suture of a tendon.

TESTICLE (TES-tih-kl): see TESTIS.

TESTICULAR CARCINOMA (tes-TIK-u-lar kar-sih-NO-mah): malignant tumor originating in a testis. An example is a SEMINOMA.

TESTIS (TES-tis): one of two paired male organs in the scrotal sac. The testes (pl.) produce sperm cells and male hormone (testosterone). Also called a testicle.

TESTOSTERONE (tes-TOS-teh-ron): a hormone that produces male secondary sex characteristics; an ANDROGEN.

THORACENTESIS (tho-rah-sen-TE-sis): surgical puncture of the chest to remove fluid; thoracocentesis.

THORACIC (tho-RAS-ik): pertaining to the chest.

THORACIC CAVITY (tho-RAS-ik KAV-ih-te): space above the abdomen that contains the heart, lungs, and other organs; the chest cavity.

THORACIC REGION (tho-RAS-ik RE-jin): backbones attached to the ribs and located in the region of the chest, between the neck and the waist.

THORACIC SURGEON (tho-RAS-ik SUR-jin): physician who operates on organs in the chest.

THORACIC VERTEBRA (tho-RAS-ik VER-teh-bra): a backbone in the region of the chest.

THORACOTOMY (tho-rah-KOT-o-me): incision of the chest.

THROAT (throt): see PHARYNX.

THROMBOCYTE (THROM-bo-sit): clotting cell; a platelet.

THROMBOLYTIC THERAPY (throm-bo-LIT-ik THER-ah-pe): treatment with drugs such as streptokinase and tPA (tissue plasminogen activator) to dissolve clots that may cause a heart attack.

THROMBOPHLEBITIS (throm-bo-fle-BI-tis): inflammation of a vein accompanied by formation of a clot.

THROMBOSIS (throm-BO-sis): abnormal condition of clot formation.

THROMBUS (THROM-bus): blood clot.

THYMOMA (thi-MO-mah): tumor (malignant) of the thymus gland.

THYMUS GLAND (THI-mus gland):   endocrine gland in the middle of the chest that produces the hormone *thymosin*. A much larger gland in children, the thymus aids the immune system by stimulating the production of white blood cells (lymphocytes).

THYROADENITIS (thi-ro-ah-de-NI-tis):   inflammation of the thyroid gland.

THYROIDECTOMY (thi-roy-DEK-to-me):   removal of the thyroid gland.

THYROID GLAND (THI-royd gland):   endocrine gland in the neck that produces hormones, which act on cells all over the body. The hormones increase the activity of cells by stimulating metabolism and the release of energy.

THYROID-STIMULATING HORMONE (THI-royd STIM-ula-ting HOR-mon):   hormone secreted by the pituitary gland to stimulate the thyroid gland to produce its hormones, such as thyroxine. Also called TSH.

THYROXINE (thi-ROK-sin):   hormone secreted by the thyroid gland. Also known as T_4.

TIBIA (TIB-e-ah):   larger of the two lower leg bones; the shin bone.

TINNITUS (TIN-ih-tus):   noise in the ears, such as ringing, roaring, or buzzing.

TISSUE (TISH-u):   groups of similar cells that work together to do a job in the body. Examples are muscle tissue, nerve tissue, and epithelial (skin) tissue.

TISSUE CAPILLARIES (TISH-u KAP-ih-lar-ez):   tiny blood vessels that lie near cells and through whose walls gases, food, and waste materials pass.

TOMOGRAPHY (to-MOG-rah-fe):   series of x-ray pictures that show an organ in depth by producing images of single tissue planes.

TONSILLECTOMY (ton-sih-LEK-to-me):   removal (excision) of a tonsil or TONSILS.

TONSILLITIS (ton-sih-LI-tis):   inflammation of the TONSILS.

TONSILS (TON-silz):   lymphatic tissue in the back of the mouth near the throat.

TRACHEA (TRAY-ke-ah):   tube that carries air from the throat to the BRONCHIAL TUBES; the windpipe.

TRACHEITIS (tray-ke-I-tis):   inflammation of the trachea.

TRACHEOSTOMY (tray-ke-OS-to-me):   opening of the trachea to the outside of the body.

TRACHEOTOMY (tray-ke-OT-o-me):   incision of the trachea.

TRANSABDOMINAL (trans-ab-DOM-ih-nal):   pertaining to across the abdomen.

TRANSGASTRIC (trans-GAS-trik):   pertaining to across the stomach.

TRANSHEPATIC (tranz-he-PAH-tik):   pertaining to across or through the liver.

TRANSURETHRAL (trans-u-RE-thral):   pertaining to across (through) the urethra. A TURP is a transurethral resection of the prostate by surgery through the urethra.

TRANSVAGINAL ULTRASOUND (tranz-VAH-jin-al UL-trah-sound):   a sound probe is placed in the vagina and ultrasound images are made of the pelvic organs (uterus and ovaries).

TRANSVERSE PLANE (trans-VERS plan):   imaginary line that divides an organ or the body into an upper and lower portion; a cross-sectional view.

TRICUSPID VALVE (tri-KUS-pid valv):   fold of tissue between the upper and lower chambers on the right side of the heart. It has three cusps or points and prevents backflow of blood into the right ATRIUM when the heart is pumping blood.

TRIGLYCERIDE (tri-GLIS-eh-ride):   fat consisting of three molecules of fatty acid and glycerol. It makes up most animal and vegetable fats and is the major lipid (fat) in blood.

TUBERCULOSIS (too-ber-ku-LO-sis):   infectious, inflammatory disease that commonly affects the lungs, although it can occur in any part of the body. It is caused by the tubercle bacillus (type of bacteria).

TYMPANIC MEMBRANE (tim-PAN-ik MEM-bran):   see EARDRUM.

TYMPANOPLASTY (tim-pan-o-PLAS-te):   surgical repair of the eardrum.

ULCER (UL-ser):   sore or defect in the surface of an organ. Ulcers are produced by destruction of tissue.

ULCERATIVE COLITIS (ul-seh-RA-TIV ko-LI-tis):   recurrent disorder marked by ULCERS in the large bowel. Along with Crohn disease, ulcerative colitis is an INFLAMMATORY BOWEL DISEASE with no known etiology (cause).

ULNA (UL-nah):   one of two lower arm bones. The ulna is located on the little finger side of the hand.

ULTRASONOGRAPHY (ul-trah-so-NOG-rah-fe):   recording of internal body structures using sound waves.

ULTRASOUND (UL-tra-sownd):   sound waves with greater frequency than can be heard by the human ear. This energy is used to detect abnormalities by beaming the waves into the body and recording echoes that reflect off tissues.

UNILATERAL (u-nih-LAT-er-al):   pertaining to one side.

UPPER GASTROINTESTINAL (GI) SERIES (UP-per gas-tro-in-TES-tin-al SER-ez):   barium is swallowed and x-ray images are taken of the esophagus, stomach and small intestine.

UREA (u-RE-ah):   chief nitrogen-containing waste that the kidney removes from the blood and eliminates from the body in urine.

UREMIA (u-RE-me-ah):   abnormal condition of excessive amounts of UREA in the bloodstream.

URETER (YOOR-eh-ter or u-RE-ter):   one of two tubes that lead from the kidney to the urinary bladder.

URETERECTOMY (u-re-ter-EK-to-me):   removal (excision) of a ureter.

URETHRA (u-RE-thrah):   tube that carries urine from the urinary bladder to the outside of the body. In males, the urethra, which is within the penis, also carries sperm from the VAS DEFERENS to the outside of the body when sperm are discharged (ejaculation).

URETHRAL STRICTURE (u-RE-thral STRIK-shur):   narrowing of the urethra.

URETHRITIS (u-re-THRI-tis):   inflammation of the urethra.

URINALYSIS (u-rih-NAL-ih-sis):   examination of urine to determine its contents.

URINARY BLADDER (UR-in-er-e BLA-der):   muscular sac that holds urine and then releases it to leave the body through the urethra.

URINARY SYSTEM (UR-in-er-e SIS-tem):   organs that produce and send urine out of the body. These organs are the kidneys, ureters, bladder, and urethra.

URINARY TRACT (UR-in-er-e trakt):   tubes and organs that carry urine from the kidney to the outside of the body.

URINE (UR-in):   fluid that is produced by the kidneys, passed through the ureters, stored in the bladder, and released from the body through the urethra.

UROLOGIST (u-ROL-o-jist):   specialist in operating on the urinary tract in males and females and on the reproductive tract in males.

UROLOGY (u-ROL-o-je): study of the urinary system in males and females and the reproductive tract in males.

UTERINE (U-ter-in): pertaining to the uterus.

UTERINE TUBES (U-ter-in tubz): see FALLOPIAN TUBES.

UTERUS (U-ter-us): muscular organ in a female that holds and provides nourishment for the developing fetus; the WOMB.

VAGINA (vah-JI-nah): muscular passageway from the uterus to the outside of the body.

VAGINITIS (vah-jih-NI-tis): inflammation of the vagina.

VARICOCELE (VAR-ih-ko-sel): swollen, twisted veins within the spermatic cord, above the testes. It produces a swelling in the scrotum that feels like a "bag of worms."

VARIX (VAH-riks): enlarged, swollen, tortuous veins (pl. varices [VAH-ri-sez]).

VAS DEFERENS (vas DEHF-or-enz): one of two tubes that carry sperm from the testes to the urethra for ejaculation.

VASCULAR (VAS-ku-lar): pertaining to blood vessels.

VASCULITIS (vas-ku-LI-tis): inflammation of blood vessels.

VASECTOMY (vas-EK-to-me): removal of the vas deferens or a portion of it so that sperm cells are prevented from becoming part of SEMEN.

VASOCONSTRICTOR (vas-o-kon-STRIK-tor): drug that narrows blood vessels, especially small arteries.

VASODILATOR (vas-o-DI-la-tor): agent that widens blood vessels.

VEIN (van): blood vessel that carries blood back to the heart from tissues of the body.

VENTRICLE (VEN-tri-kl): one of the two lower chambers of the heart. The right ventricle receives blood from the right atrium (upper chamber) and sends it to the lungs. The left ventricle receives blood from the left atrium and sends it to the body through the aorta.

VENULE (VEN-ul): small vein.

VENULITIS (ven-u-LI-tis): inflammation of a small vein.

VERTEBRA (VER-teh-brah): a backbone.

VERTEBRAE (VER-teh-bray): backbones.

VERTEBRAL (VER-teh-bral): pertaining to a backbone.

VESICAL (VES-ih-kal): pertaining to the urinary bladder (VESIC/O).

VIRUS (VI-rus): small infectious agent that can reproduce itself only when it is inside another living cell (host).

VISCERAL (VIS-er-al): pertaining to internal organs.

WOMB (woom): see UTERUS.

GLOSSARY OF WORD PARTS

Section I of this glossary is a list of **medical terminology** word parts and their **English** meanings. Section II is the reverse of that list, giving **English** meanings and their corresponding **medical terminology** word parts. If you wish to identify various combining forms, suffixes, and prefixes for the corresponding English term, check Section II.

SECTION I: MEDICAL TERMINOLOGY → ENGLISH

WORD PART	MEANING
a-, an-	no, not
ab-	away from
abdomin/o	abdomen
-ac	pertaining to
ad-	toward
aden/o	gland
adren/o	adrenal gland
-al	pertaining to
-algia	pain
alveol/o	alveolus (air sac within the lung)
amni/o	amnion (sac that surrounds the embryo)
-an	pertaining to
ana-	up, apart
an/o	anus
angi/o	vessel (blood)
ante-	before, forward
anti-	against
aort/o	aorta
append/o, appendic/o	appendix
-ar	pertaining to
arteri/o	artery
arteriol/o	small artery
arthr/o	joint
-ary	pertaining to
-ation	process, condition
aur/o	ear
axill/o	armpit
balan/o	penis
bi-	two
bi/o	life
blephar/o	eyelid
brady-	slow

bronch/o	bronchial tube
bronchiol/o	small bronchial tube
calcane/o	calcaneus (heel bone)
capillar/o	capillary
carcin/o	cancer, cancerous
cardi/o	heart
carp/o	wrist bones (carpals)
-cele	hernia
-centesis	surgical puncture to remove fluid
cephal/o	head
cerebell/o	cerebellum (posterior part of the brain)
cerebr/o	cerebrum (largest part of the brain)
cervic/o	neck
chem/o	drug, chemical
cholecyst/o	gallbladder
choledoch/o	common bile duct
chondr/o	cartilage
chron/o	time
-cision	process of cutting
cis/o	to cut
clavicul/o	clavicle (collar bone)
-coccus	bacterium (berry-shaped); pl. -cocci
coccyg/o	tailbone
col/o	colon (large intestine)
colon/o	colon
colp/o	vagina
comi/o	to care for
con-	with, together
coni/o	dust
-coniosis	abnormal condition of dust
coron/o	heart
cost/o	rib
crani/o	skull
crin/o	secrete
-crine	secretion
-crit	separation
cry/o	cold
cutane/o	skin
cyan/o	blue
cyst/o	urinary bladder
cyt/o	cell
-cyte	cell

dermat/o, derm/o	skin
dia-	through, complete
-dipsia	thirst
duoden/o	duodenum
dur/o	dura mater (outermost meningeal layer)
dys-	abnormal, bad, difficult, painful
-eal	pertaining to
ec-	out, outside
ecto-	out, outside
-ectomy	excision (resection, removal)
electr/o	electricity
-emesis	vomiting
-emia	blood condition
en-	within, in, inner
encephal/o	brain
endo-	within, in, inner
endocrin/o	endocrine glands
endometr/o, endometri/o	endometrium (inner lining of the uterus)
enter/o	intestines (usually small intestine)
epi-	above, upon
epiglott/o	epiglottis
epitheli/o	skin (surface tissue)
erythr/o	red
esophag/o	esophagus
esthesi/o	sensation
ex-, extra-	out, outside
femor/o	femur, thigh bone
fibr/o	fibrous tissue
fibul/o	fibula (smaller lower leg bone)
gastr/o	stomach
gen/o	to produce
-gen	to produce
-genesis	producing, forming
-genic	pertaining to producing, produced by
ger/o	old age
glyc/o	sugar
gnos/o	knowledge
-gram	record
-graph	instrument to record
-graphy	process of recording, to record
gynec/o	woman, female

hemat/o, hem/o	blood
hepat/o	liver
humer/o	humerus (upper arm bone)
hyper-	excessive, above
hypo-	below, deficient
hypophys/o	pituitary gland
hyster/o	uterus
-ia	condition
iatr/o	treatment
-ic	pertaining to
ile/o	ileum (third part of small intestine)
ili/o	ilium (upper part of hip bone)
in-	in, into
-ine	pertaining to
inguin/o	groin
inter-	between
intra-	within
-ior	pertaining to
isch/o	to hold back
-ism	condition, process
-ist	specialist
-itis	inflammation
jejun/o	jejunum
lapar/o	abdomen
laryng/o	larynx (voice box)
later/o	side
ligament/o	ligament
leiomy/o	smooth muscle
leuk/o	white
lip/o	fat
-listhesis	to slip, slide
lith/o	stone
-lith	stone
-logy	study of
lumb/o	loin, waist region
lymph/o	lymph
lymphaden/o	lymph nodes
lymphangi/o	lymph vessel
lys/o	separation, breakdown, destruction
-lysis	separation, breakdown, destruction

mal-	bad
-malacia	softening
mamm/o	breast
mast/o	breast
mediastin/o	mediastinum
medull/o	medulla oblongata (lower part of the brain)
-megaly	enlargement
men/o	menstruation
mening/o	meninges (membranes covering brain and spinal cord)
meta-	beyond, change
metacarp/o	metacarpals (hand bones)
metatars/o	metatarsals (foot bones)
-meter	to measure
metr/o, metri/o	uterus; to measure
-metry	measurement
-mortem	death
-motor	movement
muscul/o	muscle
my/o	muscle
myel/o	bone marrow (with -blast, -oma, -cyte, -genic)
myel/o	spinal cord (with -gram, -itis, -cele)
myos/o	muscle
myring/o	eardrum
nas/o	nose
nat/i	birth
necr/o	death
neo-	new
nephr/o	kidney
neur/o	nerve
nos/o	disease
obstetr/o	midwife
ocul/o	eye
-oid	pertaining to, resembling
-oma	tumor, mass, swelling
onc/o	tumor
oophor/o	ovary
ophthalm/o	eye
-opsy	process of viewing
opt/o	eye
or/o	mouth
orch/o	testicle, testis
orchi/o	testicle, testis
orchid/o	testicle, testis

orth/o	straight
-osis	abnormal condition
oste/o	bone
ot/o	ear
-ous	pertaining to
ovari/o	ovary
pancreat/o	pancreas
para-	beside, near, along the side of
parathyroid/o	parathyroid gland
-partum	birth
path/o	disease
-pathy	disease condition
ped/o	child
pelv/o	hip bone
per-	through
peri-	surrounding
peritone/o	peritoneum (membrane around abdominal organs)
perone/o	fibula
-pexy	fixation (surgical)
phak/o	lens of the eye
phalang/o	phalanges (finger and toe bones)
pharyng/o	pharynx, throat
-philia	attraction to
phleb/o	vein
phren/o	diaphragm
phren/o	mind
pituitar/o	pituitary gland
plas/o	formation, growth, development
-plasm	formation, growth, development
-plasty	surgical repair
-plegia	paralysis
pleur/o	pleura (membranes surrounding the lungs)
-pnea	breathing
pneum/o	air, lung
pneumon/o	lung
-poiesis	formation
post-	after, behind
pre-	before
pro-, pros-	before, forward
proct/o	anus and rectum
prostat/o	prostate gland
psych/o	mind
-ptosis	prolapse, sagging
-ptysis	spitting

pulmon/o	lung
pyel/o	renal pelvis (central section of the kidney)
radi/o	x-ray; radius (lateral lower arm bone)
re-, retro-	behind, back
rect/o	rectum
ren/o	kidney
retin/o	retina of the eye
rhabdomy/o	striated (skeletal) muscle
rheumat/o	flow, fluid
rhin/o	nose
-rrhage	bursting forth of blood
-rrhagia	bursting forth of blood
-rrhea	flow, discharge
sacr/o	sacrum
salping/o	fallopian (uterine) tube; eustachian tube
-salpinx	fallopian (uterine) tube; eustachian tube
sarc/o	flesh
scapul/o	shoulder blade (bone)
-sclerosis	hardening
-scope	instrument to view or visually examine
-scopy	process of viewing or visual examination
scrot/o	scrotal sac, scrotum
-section	to cut
sept/o	infection
septic/o	infection
-sis	condition
-somatic	pertaining to the body
son/o	sound
-spasm	constriction
spin/o	backbone, spine, vertebra
splen/o	spleen
spondyl/o	vertebra, backbone
-stasis	stop, control; place, to stand
-stat	stop, control
stern/o	sternum (breast bone)
stomat/o	mouth
-stomy	opening
sub-	under, below
sym-	with, together (use before b, p, and m)
syn-	with, together

tachy-	fast
tendin/o, ten/o	tendon
-tension	pressure
theli/o, thel/o	nipple
-therapy	treatment
-thesis	to put, to place
thorac/o	chest
thromb/o	clot
thym/o	thymus gland
thyr/o, thyroid/o, thyroaden/o	thyroid gland
tibi/o	tibia or shin bone (larger lower leg bone)
-tic	pertaining to
-tomy	incision, process of cutting
tonsill/o	tonsils
top/o	to put, place
trache/o	trachea, windpipe
trans-	across, through
tri-	three
troph/o	development, nourishment
-trophy	development, nourishment
tympan/o	eardrum
uln/o	ulna (medial lower arm bone)
ultra-	beyond
-um	structure
uni-	one
ureter/o	ureter
urethr/o	urethra
ur/o	urine, urinary tract
-uria	urine condition
uter/o	uterus
vagin/o	vagina
vas/o	vessel, vas deferens
vascul/o	blood vessel
ven/o	vein
venul/o	venule
vertebr/o	vertebra, backbone
vesic/o	urinary bladder
-y	condition, process

SECTION II: ENGLISH → MEDICAL TERMINOLOGY

MEANING	WORD PART
abdomen	abdomin/o (use with -al, -centesis)
	lapar/o (use with -scope, -scopy, -tomy)
abnormal	dys-
abnormal condition	-osis
abnormal condition of dust	-coniosis
above	epi-, hyper-
across	trans-
adrenal gland	adren/o
after	post-
against	anti-
air	pneum/o
air sac	alveol/o
along the side of	para-
alveolus	alveol/o
amnion	amni/o
anus	an/o
anus and rectum	proct/o
aorta	aort/o
apart	ana-
appendix	append/o (use with -ectomy)
	appendic/o (use with -itis)
armpit	axill/o
artery	arteri/o
attraction to	-philia
away from	ab-
back	re-, retro-
backbone	spin/o (use with -al)
	spondyl/o (use with -itis, -listhesis, -osis, -pathy)
	vertebr/o (use with -al)
bacterium (berry-shaped)	-coccus (pl. -cocci)
bad	dys-, mal-
before	ante-, pre-, pro-, pros-
behind	post-, re-, retro-
below	hypo-, sub-
beside	para-
between	inter-
beyond	meta-, ultra-
birth	nat/i, -partum

bladder (urinary)	cyst/o (use with -ic, -itis, -cele, -gram, -scopy)
	vesic/o (use with -al, -stomy, -tomy)
blood	hem/o (use with -cyte, -dialysis, -globin, -lysis, -philia, -ptysis, -rrhage, -stasis, -stat)
	hemat/o (use with -crit, -emesis, -logist, -logy, -oma, -poiesis, -salpinx, -uria)
blood condition	-emia
blood vessel	angi/o (use with -ectomy, -dysplasia, -genesis, -gram, -graphy, -oma, -plasty, -spasm)
	vas/o (use with -constriction, -dilatation, -motor)
	vascul/o (use with -ar, -itis)
blue	cyan/o
body	-somatic
bone	oste/o
bone marrow	myel/o
brain	encephal/o
breakdown	-lysis, lys/o
breast	mamm/o (use with -ary, -gram, -graphy, -plasty)
	mast/o (use with -algia, -ectomy, -itis)
breast bone	stern/o
breathing	-pnea
bronchial tube	bronch/o
bronchiole	bronchiol/o
bursting forth of blood	-rrhage, -rrhagia
calcaneus	calcane/o
cancer	carcin/o
cancerous	carcin/o
capillary	capillar/o
care for (to)	comi/o
carpals	carp/o
cartilage	chondr/o
cell	-cyte, cyt/o
cerebellum	cerebell/o
cerebrum	cerebr/o
change	meta-
chemical	chem/o
chest	thorac/o
child	ped/o
clavicle	clavicul/o
clot	thromb/o
cold	cry/o
collarbone	clavicul/o
colon	col/o (use with -ectomy, -itis, -stomy)
	colon/o (use with -pathy, -scope, -scopy)

common bile duct	choledoch/o
complete	dia-
condition	-ation, -ia, -ism, -osis, -sis, -y
constriction	-spasm
control	-stasis, -stat
cut	-cision, cis/o, -section, -tomy
death	-mortem, necr/o
deficient	hypo-
destruction	lys/o, -lysis
development	troph/o, -trophy, plas/o, -plasm
diaphragm	phren/o
difficult	dys-
discharge	-rrhea
disease	path/o, -pathy; nos/o
drug	chem/o
duodenum	duoden/o
dura mater	dur/o
dust	coni/o
dust condition	-coniosis
ear	ot/o, aur/o
eardrum	myring/o (use with -ectomy, -itis, -tomy)
	tympan/o (use with -ic, -metry, -plasty)
electricity	electr/o
endocrine gland	endocrin/o
endometrium	endometri/o
enlargement	-megaly
epiglottis	epiglott/o
esophagus	esophag/o
eustachian tube	salping/o, -salpinx
excessive	hyper-
excision	-ectomy
eye	ocul/o (use with -ar, -facial, -motor)
	ophthalm/o (use with -ia, -ic, -logist, -logy, -pathy, -plasty, -plegia, -scope, -scopy)
	opt/o (use with -ic, -metrist)
eyelid	blephar/o
fallopian tube	salping/o, -salpinx
fast	tachy-
fat	lip/o
female	gynec/o
femur	femor/o

fibrous tissue	fibr/o
fibula	fibul/o, perone/o
fixation (surgical)	-pexy
flesh	sarc/o
flow	-rrhea, rheumat/o
fluid	rheumat/o
foot bones	metatars/o
formation	plas/o, -plasm, -poiesis, -genesis
forward	ante-, pro-, pros-
gallbladder	cholecyst/o
gland	aden/o
groin	inguin/o
growth	plas/o, -plasm
hand bones	metacarp/o
hardening	-sclerosis
head	cephal/o
heart	cardi/o (use with -ac, -graphy, -logy, -logist, -megaly, -pathy, -vascular)
	coron/o (use with -ary)
heel bone	calcane/o
hernia	-cele
hip bone	pelv/o
hold back (to)	isch/o
humerus	humer/o
ileum	ile/o
ilium	ili/o
in, into	in-, en-, endo-
incision	-tomy, -section
infection	sept/o, septic/o
inflammation	-itis
inner	en-, endo-
instrument to record	-graph
instrument to view	-scope
intestines (small)	enter/o
jejunum	jejun/o
joint	arthr/o
kidney	nephr/o (use with -algia, -ectomy, -ic, -itis, -lith, -megaly, -oma, -osis, -pathy, -ptosis, -sclerosis, -stomy, -tomy)
	ren/o (use with -al, -gram)

kidney (central section)	pyel/o
knowledge	gnos/o
larynx	laryng/o
lens of the eye	phak/o
life	bi/o
ligament	ligament/o
liver	hepat/o
loin	lumb/o
lung	pneum/o (use with -coccus, -coniosis, -thorax)
	pneumon/o (use with -ectomy, -ia, -ic, -itis, -pathy)
	pulmon/o (use with -ary)
lymph	lymph/o
lymph node	lymphaden/o
lymph vessel	lymphangi/o
mass	-oma
measure (to)	metr/o, -meter, -metry
mediastinum	mediastin/o
medulla oblongata	medull/o
meninges	mening/o
menstruation	men/o
metacarpals	metacarp/o
metatarsals	metatars/o
midwife	obstetr/o
mind	psych/o, phren/o
mouth	or/o (use with -al)
	stomat/o (use with -itis)
movement	-motor
muscle	muscul/o (use with -ar, -skeletal)
	myos/o (use with -itis)
	my/o (use with -algia, -ectomy, -oma, -gram, -neural)
near	para-
neck	cervic/o
nerve	neur/o
new	neo-
nipple	theli/o, thel/o
no, not	a-, an-
nose	nas/o (use with -al)
	rhin/o (use with -itis, -rrhea, -plasty)
nourishment	troph/o, -trophy
old age	ger/o
one	uni-

opening	-stomy
out, outside	ec-, ecto-, ex-, extra-
ovary	oophor/o (use with -itis, -ectomy, -pexy, -plasty, -tomy)
	ovari/o (use with -an)
pain	-algia
painful	dys-
pancreas	pancreat/o
paralysis	-plegia
parathyroid gland	parathyroid/o
pelvis	pelv/o
pelvis (renal)	pyel/o
penis	balan/o
peritoneum	peritone/o
pertaining to	-ac, -al, -an, -ar, -ary, -eal, -ic, -ine, -ior, -oid, -ous, -tic
pertaining to the body	-somatic
phalanges	phalang/o
pharynx	pharyng/o
pituitary gland	hypophys/o, pituitar/o
place	top/o; -stasis
pleura	pleur/o
pressure	-tension
process	-ation, -ism, -y
process of cutting	-cision, -tomy, -section
process of recording	-graphy
process of viewing	-opsy, -scopy
produce (to)	-gen, gen/o
produced by	-genic
producing	-genic, -genesis
prolapse	-ptosis
prostate gland	prostat/o
puncture to remove fluid	-centesis
put, place (to)	top/o, -thesis
radius (lower arm bone)	radi/o
record	-gram
recording (process)	-graphy
rectum	rect/o
red	erythr/o
removal	-ectomy
renal pelvis	pyel/o
repair	-plasty
resection	-ectomy
resembling	-oid
retina of the eye	retin/o
rib	cost/o

sacrum	sacr/o
sagging	-ptosis
scapula	scapul/o
scrotum, scrotal sac	scrot/o
secrete, secretion	-crine, crin/o
sensation	esthesi/o
separation	-crit, -lysis, lys/o
shin bone	tibi/o
shoulder blade	scapul/o
side	later/o
skin	cutane/o (use with -ous)
	derm/o (use with -al),dermat/o (use with -itis, -logy, -osis)
	epitheli/o (use with -al)
skull	crani/o
slide	-listhesis
slip (to)	-listhesis
slow	brady-
small artery	arteriol/o
small bronchial tube	bronchiol/o
small intestine	enter/o
smooth muscle	leiomy/o
softening	-malacia
sound	son/o
specialist	-ist
spinal cord	myel/o
spine	spin/o
spitting	-ptysis
spleen	splen/o
stand (to)	-stasis
sternum	stern/o
stomach	gastr/o
stone	lith/o, -lith
stop	-stasis, -stat
straight	orth/o
striated (skeletal) muscle	rhabdomy/o
structure	-um
study of	-logy
sugar	glyc/o
surgical puncture to remove fluid	-centesis
surgical repair	-plasty
surrounding	peri-
swelling	-oma

tailbone	coccyg/o
tendon	tendin/o, ten/o
testicle, testis	orch/o, orchi/o, orchid/o
thigh bone	femor/o
thirst	-dipsia
throat	pharyng/o
three	tri-
through	dia-, per-, trans-
thymus gland	thym/o
thyroid gland	thyr/o, thyroid/o, thyroaden/o
tibia	tibi/o
time	chron/o
together	con-, syn-, sym-
tonsil	tonsill/o
toward	ad-
trachea	trache/o
treatment	iatr/o, -therapy
tumor	-oma, onc/o
two	bi-
ulna	uln/o
under	hypo-, sub-
up	ana-
upon	epi-
ureter	ureter/o
urethra	urethr/o
urinary bladder	cyst/o, vesic/o
urinary tract	ur/o
urine	ur/o
urine condition	-uria
uterine tube	salping/o
uterus	hyster/o (use with -ectomy, -graphy, -gram)
	metr/o (use with -itis, -rrhagia), metri/o
	metri/o (use with -al)
	uter/o (use with -ine)
uterus (inner lining)	endometr/o, endometri/o
vagina	colp/o (use with -pexy, -plasty, -scope, -scopy, -tomy)
	vagin/o (use with -al, -itis)
vas deferens	vas/o
vein	phleb/o (use with -ectomy, -itis, -lith, -thrombosis, -tomy)
	ven/o (use with -ous, -gram)
venule	venul/o
vertebra	spin/o (use with -al)
	spondyl/o (use with -itis, -listhesis, -osis, -pathy)
	vertebr/o (use with -al)

vessel	angi/o (use with -ectomy, -dysplasia, -genesis, -gram, -graphy, -oma, -plasty, -spasm)
	vas/o (use with -constriction, -dilation, -motor)
	vascul/o (use with -ar, -itis)
view (to)	-opsy
visual examination	-scopy
voice box	laryng/o
vomiting	-emesis
waist region	lumb/o
white	leuk/o
windpipe	trache/o
with	con-, syn-, sym-
within	en-, endo-, intra-
woman	gynec/o
wrist bones	carp/o
x-ray	radi/o

GLOSSARY OF ENGLISH → SPANISH TERMS

Here is a list of English → Spanish terms that will help you communicate with Spanish-speaking patients in offices, hospitals, and other medical settings. It includes parts of the body and other medical terms as well.

abdomen	abdomen (ahb-**DOH**-mehn)
acne	acné (ahk-**NEH**)
acoustic	acústico (ah-**KOOS**-tee-ko)
adenoid	adenoide (ah-deh-**NOH**-ee-deh)
amebic	amébico (ah-**MEH**-bee-ko)
analgesic	analgésico (ah-nahl-**HEH**-see-koh)
anemia	anemia (ah-**NEH**-mee-ah)
anesthesia	anestesia (ah-nehs-**TEH**-see-ah)
angina	angina (ahn-**HEE**-na)
angioma	angioma (ahn-hee-**OH**-mah)
ankle	tobillo (toh-**BEE**-yoh)
antacid	antiácido (ahn-tee-**AH**-see-doh)
antiarrhythmic	antiarritmia (ahn-tee-ah-**REET**-mee-ah)
antibiotic	antibiótico (ahn-tee-bee-**OH**-tee-koh)
anticonvulsant	anticonvulsivo (ahn-tee-kohn-bool-**SEE**-boh)
antidiarrheal	antidiarrético (ahn-tee-dee-ah-**RHEH**-tee-koh)
antiemetic	antiemético (ahn-tee-eh-**MEH**-tee-koh)
antiepileptic	antiepiléptico (ahn-tee-eh-pee-**LEHP**-tee-koh)
antihistamine	antihistamínico (ahn-tee-ees-tah-**MEE**-nee-koh)
antiviral	antivirus (ahn-tee-**BEE**-roos)
anus	ano (**AH**-no)
appendix	apéndice (ah-**PEHN**-dee-seh)
armpit	axila (ahx-**EE**-lah)
arteriogram	arteriograma (ahr-teh-ree-oh-**GRAH**-mah)
arthritis	artritis (ahr-**TREE**-tees)
asthma	asma (**AHS**-mah)
bacteria	bacteria (bahk-**TEH**-ree-ah)
barbiturates	barbitúricos (bahr-bee-**TOO**-ree-kohs)
birthmark	lunar (loo-**NAHR**)
bleeding	sangrando (sahn-**GRAHN**-do)
blood	sangre (**SAHN**-greh)
blood count	biometría hemática (bee-oh-meh-**TREE**-ah eh-**MAH**-tee-kah)
bradycardia	bradicardia (brah-dee-**KAHR**-dee-ah)
brain	cerebro (seh-**REH**-bro)
breast/chest	seno (**SEH**-noh), pecho (**PEH**-choh)
bronchial tube	bronquio (**BROHN**-kee-oh)
bronchitis	bronquitis (brohn-**KEE**-tees)
bruises	moretones (moh-reh-**TOHN**-ehs)
burn	quemadura (keh-mah-**DOO**-rah)

calf	pantorrilla (pahn-toh-**REE**-yah)
callus	callo (**KAH**-yoh)
calm	calma (**KAHL**-mah)
cardiac	cardiaco (kahr-**DEE**-ah-koh)
cataract	catarata (kah-tah-**RAH**-tah)
cervix	cuello uterino (**KOO**-eh-joh oo-teh-**REE**-noh), cerviz (**SERH**-beex)
chancre	chancro (**CHAHN**-kroh)
cheek	mejilla (meh-**HEE**-yah)
chemotherapy	quimioterapia (kee-mee-oh-teh-**RAH**-pee-ah)
chin	barbilla (bar-**BEE**-ya)
cholesterol	colesterol (koh-lehs-teh-**ROHL**)
cirrhosis	cirrosis (see-**RROH**-sees)
claustrophobia	claustrofobia (klah-oos-troh-**FOH**-bee-ah)
coagulation	coagulación (koh-ah-goo-lah-see-**OHN**)
collar bone	clavícula (klah-**VEE**-kuh-la)
colon	colón (**KOH**-lohn)
constipation	estreñimiento (ehs-treh-nyee-mee-**EHN**-toh)
cortisone	cortisona (kohr-tee-**SOH**-nah)
cough	tos (tohs)
cyanotic	cianótico (see-ah-**NOH**-tee-ko)
decongestants	descongestionantes (dehs-kohn-hehs-tee-oh-**NAHN**-tehs)
dehydrated	deshidratado (deh-see-drah-**TAH**-do)
delirious	delirio (deh-**LEE**-ree-oh)
depressed	deprimido (deh-pree-**MEE**-doh)
diabetes	diabetes (dee-ah-**BEH**-tehs)
diarrhea	diarrea (dee-ah-**RREH**-ah)
digitalis	digitales (dee-hee-**TAH**-les)
ear (inner)	oído (oh-**EE**-do)
ear (outer)	oreja (oh-**REH**-hah)
ecchymosis	equimosis (eh-kee-**MOH**-sees)
eczema	eccema (ehk-**SEH**-mah)
elbow	codo (**KOH**-doh)
embolism	embolismo (ehm-boh-**LEES**-moh)
emetic	emético (eh-**MEH**-tee-koh)
enteritis	enteritis (ehn-teh-**REE**-tees)
epilepsy	epilepsia (eh-pee-**LEHP**-seeah)
euphoric	eufórico (eh-oo-**FOH**-ree-koh)
exudate	exudado (ehk-soo-**DAH**-doh)
eye	ojo (**OH**-hoh)
eyebrow	ceja (**SEH**-hah)
eyelash	pestaña (pehs-**TAH**-nyah)
eyelids	párpados (**PAHR**-pah-dohs)

fibroid	fibroide (fee-**BROY**-deh)
finger	dedo (**DEH**-doh)
fingernail	uña (**OO**-nyah)
fist	puño (**POO**-nyoh)
fistula	fistula (**FEES**-too-lah)
foot	pié (pee-**EH**)
forearm	antebrazo (an-teh-**BRAH**-zoh)
forehead	frente (**FREN**-teh)
fungus	hongos (**OHN**-gohs)
gallbladder	vesícula biliar (beh-**SEE**-koo-lah bee-lee-**AHR**)
gangrene	gangrena (gahn-**GREH**-nah)
gastroenteritis	gastroenteritis (gahs-troh-ehn-teh-**REE**-tees)
gastroenterology	gastroenterología (gahs-troh-ehn-teh-roh-loh-**HEE**-ah)
genital organs	órganos genitales (**ORH**-gah-nohs heh-nee-**TAH**-lehs)
glaucoma	glaucoma (glah-oo-**KOH**-mah)
groin	ingle (**EEN**-gleh)
gums	encías (ehn-**SEE**-ahs)
gynecologist	ginecólogo (hee-neh-**KOH**-loh-goh)
hair	cabello (kah-**BEH**-yoh)
hand	mano (**MAH**-noh)
heart	corazón (koh-rah-**SOHN**)
hematology	hematología (eh-mah-toh-loh-**HEE**-ah)
hematoma	hematoma (eh-mah-**TOH**-ma)
hemolysis	hemólisis (eh-**MOH**-lee-sees)
hemorrhage	hemorragia (eh-moh-**RRAH**-heeah)
hepatitis	hepatitis (eh-pah-**TEE**-tees)
hernia	hernia (**EHR**-neeah)
hip	cadera (kah-**DEH**-rah)
hypertension	hipertensión (ee-pehr-tehn-see-**OHN**)
icteric	ictérico (eek-**TEH**-ree-koh)
infection	infección (een-fehk-see-**OHN**)
inflammation	inflamación (een-flah-mah-see-**OHN**)
insulin	insulina (een-soo-**LEE**-nah)
intestine	intestino (een-tes-**TEE**-noh)
intramuscular	intramuscular (een-trah-moos-koo-**LAHR**)
intravenous	intravenoso (een-trah-beh-**NOH**-soh)
irradiate	irradiar (ee-rrhah-dee-**AHR**)
jaw	mandívula (mahn-**DEE**-boo-lah)
kidney	riñón (ree-**NYON**)
knee	rodilla (ro-**DEE**-yah)

laparoscopy	laparoscopia (lah-pah-rohs-**KOH**-peeah)
laryngitis	laringitis (lah-reen-**HEE**-tees)
laxative	laxante (lahx-**AHN**-teh)
left	izquierdo (ees-kee-**EHR**-doh)
leg	pierna (pee-**EHR**-nah)
ligament	ligamento (lee-gah-**MEHN**-toh)
lingual	lingual (leen-**GUAHL**)
lip	labio (**LAH**-bee-oh)
lithium	litio (**LEE**-tee-oh)
liver	hígado (**EE**-gah-doh)
low cholesterol	poca colesterol (**POH**-kah koh-lehs-teh-**RHOL**)
low fat	poca grasa (**POH**-kah **GRAH**-sah)
low sodium	poca sal (**POH**-kah sahl)
lung	pulmón (pool-**MOHN**)
meningitis	meningitis (meh-neen-**HEE**-tees)
morphine	morfina (mohr-**FEE**-nah)
mouth	boca (**BOH**-kah)
muscle	músculo (**MOOS**-koo-loh)
narcotics	narcóticos (nahr-**KOH**-tee-kohs)
nasal	nasal (nah-**SAHL**)
nausea	náusea (**NAH**-oo-seh-ah)
navel	ombligo (ohm-**BLEE**-goh)
neck	cuello (koo-**EH**-yoh)
neonatal	neonatal (neh-oh-nah-**TAHL**)
nephrologist	nefrólogo (nehp-**PHROH**-lo-goh)
nephrology	nefrología (neh-phroh-lo-**HEEAH**)
nervous	nervioso (nehr-bee-**OH**-soh)
neurotic	neurótico (neh-oo-**ROH**-tee-koh)
nipple	pezón (peh-**SOHN**)
nitroglycerin	nitroglicerina (nee-troh-glee-seh-**REE**-nah)
nose	nariz (nah-**REES**)
nostrils	fosas nasales (foh-**SAHS** na-**SAH**-lehs)
Novocain	novocaína (noh-boh-kah-**EE**-nah)
nuclear medicine	medicina nuclear (meh-dee-**SEE**-nah **NOO**-kleh-ahr)
obstetrics	obstetricia (ohbs-tee-**TREE**-see-ah)
oncology	oncología (ohn-koh-loh-**HEE**-ah)
ophthalmic	oftálmico (ohf-**TAHL**-mee-koh)
ophthalmology	oftalmología (ohf-tahl-moh-loh-**HEE**-ah)
optic	óptico (**OHP**-tee-koh)
orthopedics	ortopédia (ohr-toh-**PEH**-dee-ah)
orthopedic surgeon	cirujano ortopéico (see-roo-**HAH**-noh ohr-toh-**PEH**-dee-koh)

otic	otico (**OH**-tee-koh)
ovary	ovario (oh-**BAH**-ree-oh)
palate	paladar (pah-lah-**DAHR**)
palpation	palpación (pahl-pah-see-**OHN**)
palpitation	palpitación (pahl-pee-tah-see-**OHN**)
pancreas	páncreas (**PAHN**-kreh-ahs)
pancreatitis	pancreatitis (pahn-kreh-ah-**TEE**-tees)
paralytic	paralítico (pah-rah-**LEE**-tee-koh)
pathogen	patogen (pah-toh-**HEHN**)
pathological	patológico (pah-toh-**LOH**-hee-koh)
pathology	patología (pah-toh-loh-**HEE**-ah)
pediatrics	pediatría (peh-dee-ah-**TREE**-ah)
pelvis	pelvis (**PEHL**-bees)
penis	pene (**PEH**-neh), miembro (mee-**EHM**-broh)
pneumonia	pulmonía/neumonía (pool-moh-**NEE**-ah/neh-oo-moh-**NEE**-ah)
pruritic	prurito (proo-**REE**-toh)
psychiatrist	psiquiatra (see-kee-**AH**-trah)
psychiatry	psiquiatria (see-kee-**AH**-tree-ah)
psychologist	psicólogo (see-**KOH**-loh-goh)
psoriasis	soriasis (soh-ree-**AH**-sees)
pubic	púbico (**POO**-bee-koh)
pyorrhea	piorrea (pee-oh-**RREH**-ah)
radiologist	radiologo (rah-dee-**OH**-loh-goh)
radiology	radiología (rah-dee-oh-loh-**HEEAH**)
rectum	recto (**REHK**-toh)
rheumatic	reumático (reh-oo-**MAH**-tee-koh)
rib	costilla (kohs-**TEE**-yah)
right	derecho (deh-**REH**-choh)
roseola	roseóla (roh-seh-**OH**-lah)
rubella	rubeóla (roo-beh-**OH**-lah)
scalp	cuero cabelludo (**KOO**-eh-roh kah-beh-**YOO**-doh)
sebaceous	sebáceo (seh-**BAH**-seh-oh)
sedatives	sedativos/sedantes (seh-dah-**TEE**-bohs/seh-**DAHN**-tehs)
shin	espinilla (ehs-pee-**NEE**-yah)
shoulder	hombro (**OHM**-bro)
skin	piel (pee-**EHL**)
skull	cráneo (**KRAH**-ne-oh)
spinal column	columna vertebral (koh-**LUHM**-nah behr-teh-**BRAHL**)
spleen	bazo (**BAH**-zoh), esplín (ehs-**PLEEN**)
stethoscope	estetoscópio (ehs-teh-tohs-**KOH**-pee-oh)
stomach	estómago (ehs-**TOH**-mah-goh)
stool sample	muestra de excremento (moo-**EHS**-trah deh ehs-kreh-**MENH**-toh)
straight	derecho (deh-**REH**-choh)

subaxillary	subaxilar (soob-**AHX**-ee-lahr)
subcutaneous	subcutáneo (soob-koo-**TAH**-neh-oh)
sublingual	sublingual (soob-**LEEN**-goo-ahl)
substernal	subesternal (soob-ehs-**TEHR**-nahl)
surgeon	cirujano (see-roo-**HAH**-noh)
surgery	cirugía (see-roo-**HEE**-ah)
symptoms	síntomas (**SEEN**-toh-mahs)
syncope	síncope (**SEEN**-koh-peh)
systole	sístole (**SEES**-toh-leh)
teeth	dientes (dee-**EHN**-tehs)
temple	sien (see-**EHN**)
testicles	testículos (tehs-**TEE**-koo-lohs)
tetanus	tétano (**TEH**-tah-noh)
therapy	terapia (teh-**RAH**-pee-ah)
thigh	muslo (**MOOS**-loh)
throat	garganta (gahr-**GAHN**-tah)
thyroid	tiroide (tee-**ROY**-deh)
toes	dedos (**DEH**-dos), del pié (dehl **PEE**-eh)
tongue	lengua (**LEHN**-goo-ah)
tonsillitis	tonsilitis/amigdalitis (tohn-see-**LEE**-tees/ah-meeg-dah-**LEE**-tees)
tonsils	amígdalas (ah-**MEEG**-da-las)
ulcer	úlcera (**OOL**-seh-rah)
ulnar	ulnar (**OOL**-nahr)
ultrasound	ultrasonido (ool-trah-soh-**NEE**-doh)
uremia	uremia (oo-**REH**-mee-ah)
urinary bladder	vejiga (beh-**HEE**-gah)
urine	orina (oh-**REE**-nah)
urticaria	urticaria (oor-tee-**KAH**-ree-ah)
uterus	útero (**OO**-teh-roh)
uvula	úvula (**OO**-boo-lah)
vaginitis	vaginitis (bah-hee-**NEE**-tees)
vagus	vago (**BAH**-goh)
valve	válvula (**BAHL**-boo-lah)
varicocele	varicocéle (bah-ree-koh-**SEH**-leh)
vertigo	vértigo (**BEHR**-tee-goh)
waist	cintura (sin-**TOO**-rah)
womb	vientre (bee-**EHN**-treh)
wrist	muñeca (moo-**NYEH**-kah)
x-rays	rayos equis (rah-**YOHS EH**-kees)
zygomatic	cigomático (see-goh-**MAH**-tee-koh)

INDEX

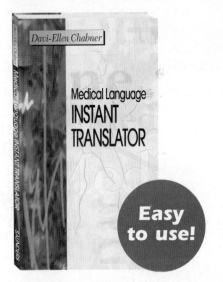